New and Expanded Neuropsychosocial Concepts Complementary to Llorens' Developmental Theory

This book analyzes and suggests an expansion of Llorens' developmental theory of occupational therapy, applying these concepts in a final schematic model for use by occupational therapists, occupational scientists, and others involved in occupational tasks, relationships, and activities. The book then uses the International Classification of Functioning in a context of health promotion and disease prevention to relate the expanded theory to psychosocial, cognitive, and sensorimotor correlates in preterm infants and their families in the neonatal intensive care unit and after discharge to the home environment. Last, it provides an NICU infant case illustration on the Developmental Analysis, Evaluation, and Intervention Schedule.

The major theme of this book focuses upon expanding the psychological, neurophysiological, and sociological aspects of Llorens' developmental theory for a person-occupation-environment based practice and research. The book will then correlate these concepts with current terminology from the World Health Organization, and specialized knowledge and skills in the neonatal intensive care unit.

This book was published as a special issue of *Occupational Therapy in Mental Health*.

Dr. La Corte's current affiliations are as follows: PhD Candidate in the College of Health Science, Walden University; Primary Children's Hospital, Salt Lake City, Utah; Private Practice; Adjunct Faculty, Division of Occupational Therapy, University of Utah, Salt Lake City, Utah. She has taught multiple courses on infant development, and has published case study and poster presentation abstracts. Further to this, she has provided occupational therapy services in the primary care setting in various NICUs, and at Aviano Air Force Base, Aviano, Italy, for developmental screening of all newborn infants and to support infant, mother, and family co-occupations.

New and Expanded Neuropsychosocial Concepts Complementary to Llorens' Developmental Theory

Achieving Growth and Development through Occupation for Neonatal Infants and their Families

Lynne F. La Corte

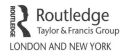
Routledge
Taylor & Francis Group

LONDON AND NEW YORK

First published 2009 by Routledge
2 Park Square, Milton Park, Abingdon, Oxon, OX14 4RN

Simultaneously published in the USA and Canada
by Routledge
270 Madison Avenue, New York, NY 10016

Routledge is an imprint of the Taylor & Francis Group, an informa business

© 2009 Lynne F. La Corte

Typeset in Times by Value Chain, India
Printed and bound in Great Britain by CPI Rowe, Chippenham, Wiltshire

British Library Cataloguing in Publication Data
A catalogue record for this book is available from the British Library

ISBN10: 0-7890-3468-9 (hbk)
ISBN10: 0-7890-3469-7 (pbk)
ISBN13: 978-0-7890-3468-7 (hbk)
ISBN13: 978-0-7890-3469-4 (pbk)

CONTENTS

LIST OF TABLES

LIST OF FIGURES

This book is dedicated to the life and work of
Lela A. Llorens, Ph.D., OTR, FAOTA

Foreword

It is distinctly gratifying for a teacher/mentor/author to have her work appreciated and utilized by her students in their practice. In this case, my former student and current colleague/mentee has not only utilized my work in practice, she has continued to study the work and has now expanded and extended it in both breadth and depth. In this issue, Lynne F. La Corte, OTD, MHS, presents further analysis of a developmental theory for health promotion, dysfunction/disability prevention, therapy, and rehabilitation. The original work on which this volume is based has stood the test of time as theory and frame of reference (Crepeau, Cohn, & Schell, 2003). Dr. La Corte has brought a fresh look and point of view as well as incredible depth to the neurophysiological aspects of the theory and application of developmental theory in the evaluation and therapeutic management of infants in the Neonatal Intensive Care Unit.

It is still my belief, as stated in the preface of *Application of a Developmental Theory for Health and Rehabilitation* (Llorens, 1976), that Occupational Therapy is a problem-solving process for the treatment and training of the ill and disabled for restoration of function, and intervention in the lives of the well and able for prevention of disability and maintenance of health. Those who receive services from occupational therapists require individualized treatment for the problems that they present. No two clients can be treated exactly the same even if they present with the same diagnosis. Some of the differences related to their care may be dictated by age, gender, life role expectations, cultural background, environmental requirements, physical involvement, and psychological temperament. These variables along with the medical and/or health conditions with which the person presents will have an effect on the growing individual at a specific time in their life span in which the condition to be rectified occurs. We know that interventions that include activities, occupations, and interpersonal interaction can assist in the facilitation of functional outcomes.

The practice of occupational therapy is complex. Its theoretical foundations are based upon the developing science of occupation and the established biological, psychological, and social sciences. The art of practice requires the therapist to analyze and utilize knowledge from all such fields in the process of determining the occupational problem. Collaboratively, with the client and/or parent or guardian, the therapist then plans a course of therapy that will resolve the occupational dilemma in the direction of appropriate functional outcomes.

According to a statement that appears in the introduction to *Occupational Therapy Sequential Client Care Record Manual* (Llorens, 1982), the successful practice of occupational therapy is dependent upon the occupational therapist's knowledge of the person, appropriate activities and occupations, and effective utilization of interpersonal interaction to effect personal growth. The analysis and synthesis of this knowledge for application to help individual clients solve problems encountered or anticipated in their daily lives is the essence of occupational therapy practice. "Successful practice requires the therapist to assess acquired knowledge, evaluate client behavior and performance, and plan and implement treatment or training to maintain, restore, or improve the client's ability to function" (Llorens, 1982, p. 1). Parameters along which knowledge of the human may be assessed include neurological, physiological, physical, psychological, social, environmental, and intellectual areas of development. Abilities in the areas of daily living and social language skills and developmental occupations and ego-adaptive skills may also be assessed. Information gained in initial and continuing assessment is used in the determination of objectives and goals to be attained as outcomes of therapy.

With a focus on cerebral palsy and learning disorders purportedly resulting from birth trauma, Dr. La Corte has used the Llorens developmental theory and framework to guide her work. She has expanded the original work to include more in-depth knowledge of neurological concepts and has extended the revision to include health promotion, disease/disability prevention, rehabilitation, and therapy.

Dr. La Corte provides the reader with an historical and contemporary perspective of analysis and application of this developmental theory. Dr. La Corte's extensive experience gained from working with infants, children, and their parents have informed the power of her observations. An impressive depth of knowledge of how incoming information is processed by the nervous system has provided a substantial degree of sophistication to Dr. La Corte's analysis, expansion, and extension of the original work.

Lela A. Llorens, PhD, OTR, FAOTA
Professor Emeritus, San Jose State University, San Jose, CA
Adjunct Professor, University of Southern California,
Los Angeles, CA
Consultant, Occupational Therapy and Gerontology

REFERENCES

Crepeau, E. B., Cohn, E. S., & Schell, B. A. B. (2003). *Willard & Spackman's occupational therapy*. Philadelphia: Lippincott, Williams & Wilkins.

Llorens, L. A. (1976). *Application of a developmental therapy*. Bethesda, MD: American Occupational Therapy Association.

Llorens, L. A. (1982). *Occupational therapy sequential client care record manual*. Laurel, MD: Ramsco Publishing.

Preface

Understanding the role of adaptation in the development of occupational beings throughout the life span provides a great deal of insight about the variation humans possess for change. As such, the central nervous system processes enormous amounts of perceptual data as purpose and intent are drawn from ones relationships and environmental activities. An awareness of animal models and their linkage to human occupational engagement promotes understanding of adaptive change processes.

Lynne F. La Corte, OTD, MHS

New and Expanded Neuropsychosocial Concepts Complementary to Llorens' Developmental Theory: Achieving Growth and Development through Occupation for Neonatal Infants and their Families

Lynne F. La Corte, OTD, MHS

INTRODUCTION

Cerebral palsy is the most common physical disability in childhood (Surveillance of Cerebral Palsy in Europe (SCPE), 2002; Winter, Autry, Boyle, & Yeargin-Allsopp, 2002). Epidemiological studies of industrialized countries indicate that cerebral palsy occurs in 2.0 to 2.5 per 1000 live births (Hagberg, Hagberg, Beckung, & Uvebrant, 2001; Paneth & Kiely, 1984; Parkes, Dolk, Hill, & Pattenden, 2001). CP is defined as a movement impairment ranging from mild to severe (Bax et al., 2005; Bobath, 1954; Nelson, 2001) and occurs through social, physical, and environmental causal pathways that result in a brain lesion sometime during the ante-, peri-, or post-natal period of birth (Stanley, Blair, & Alberman, 2000).

Advances in medical technology over the past 20 years have led to a marked decrease in infant mortality (Bennett & Scott, 1997; Hagberg et al., 2001). As a result, there has been a consistent rise in preterm and extremely preterm survival rates during this same time period (Hagberg et al., 2001; Reddihough & Collins, 2003; Robertson, Svenson, & Joffres, 1998). Specifically, between 8–10% of all very low birth weight (VLBW) infants (<1500 grams) and 25% of all extremely low birth weight (ELBW) infants (<1000 grams) will develop cerebral palsy (CP) and/or sensory-neural impairments

(Wilson-Costello, Friedman, Minich, Fanaroff, & Hack, 2005), with trends stabilizing since the mid 1990s (Robertson, Watt, & Yasui, 2007). Motor, cognitive, behavioral, and perceptual impairments significantly impact learning and educational achievement, psychosocial well-being and relationships, and daily self-care activities (Bennett & Scott, 1997; Bhutta, Cleves, Casey, Cradock, & Annand, 2002; Majnemer, 1998; Majnemer & Rosenblatt, 1995; Sajaniemi et al., 2001).

For ELBW and VLBW children and their families, a biopsychosocial model (Mosey, 1974) provides a conceptual framework to explain, measure, and support an infant and their family's intrinsic and extrinsic drives for competence and mastery within the context of sociocultural adaptation to the environmental demands of a neonatal intensive care unit (NICU) (Gilfoyle, Grady, & Moore, 1990; Llorens, 1970, 1976, 1977a; Schultz & Schkade, 1992a, 1992b). To understand the needs of infants and their families in the NICU, a thorough understanding of growth and development is imperative. Several major theorists have contributed models of growth and development as the human organism strives to acquire mastery and competence in the human adaptation process, such as Ayres (1972), Bandura (1977a, 1977b), Bronfenbrenner (1979), Bruner (1966, 1976), Erikson (1964), Freud (1938), Gesell & Ilg (1949), Grant (1963), Hall (1954), Havighurst (1972), Mosey (1986), Papalia, Olds, & Feldman (2001), Pearce & Newton (1963), Peck and Havighurst (1960), and Piaget (1952).

In her theory entitled *The Developmental Theory of Occupational Therapy* (also known as *Facilitating Growth and Development...*), Llorens (1970) captured the essence of many of these major theorists' constructs pertaining to the development of mastery and competence in everyday occupations throughout the lifespan. In the early detection of cerebral palsy, developmental coordination and sensory processing disorders resulting from NICU sequelae, the Llorens model provides a guiding framework for the explanatory and predictive aspects of the theoretical application to practice. The explanatory aspects of Llorens' theory provide continuums of occupational function to dysfunction that allow the occupational therapist and scientist to seek out and identify infant and family needs. The predictive value of Llorens' theory provides postulates regarding occupational change for the application of meaningful and purposeful activities and relationships for adaptive infant and family occupation in the NICU.

The purpose of this book is to review, update, and expand the Developmental Theory of Occupational Therapy for application in relationship to health promotion, disease prevention, therapy, and rehabilitation. In particular, the author applies the expanded schematic in the NICU.

This book provides four separate but interrelated components. In Part 1, the author reviews and examines Llorens' thesis, theoretical premises, and schematic model. She then analyzes, evaluates, and recommends new concepts and theorists for model expansion of the *Developmental Theory of Occupational Therapy* (Llorens, 1970). In Part 2, the author analyzes the concept of central pattern generators to explain Llorens' (1970) prediction about why occupational therapists use activities (occupation) and relationships to facilitate adaptive growth and development. The author posits that the sensorimotor process of *occupational physiology* serves as the adaptive change mechanism in central pattern generation to explain the inherent value of occupation as purposeful activities and relationships. In Part 3, the author applies the recommendations for expansion from Parts 1 and 2 sections to the *Developmental Theory of Occupational Therapy*. This application expands Llorens' schematic model to include revisions, modifications, the incorporation of additional theorists, and current occupational theoretical concepts. A revision of Llorens' theoretical premises reflect current concepts of health promotion, disease prevention, rehabilitation, and therapy. Llorens' expanded schematic and theoretical premises provide a basis for the application of occupational therapy practice and process models within the physical and sociocultural environment of the NICU. In Part 4, the author presents a modified version of Llorens' (1977b) developmental analysis, evaluation, and intervention schedule (DAEIS), with a case illustration utilizing Llorens' expanded theory.

PART 1: THEORY ANALYSIS AND NEW CONCEPTS

The goal of Part 1 of this book is to analyze Llorens' theoretical model and to make recommendations for its expansion. First, Llorens' original 1970 thesis, premises, and schematic illustrate the Llorens theory, along with the author's interpretation of same. Tracing the model's history to more recent additions and changes made in 1976 and 1991 from the original version in 1970 analyzes theory development over a 20-year period.

Second, an evaluation of the model's most recent changes (Llorens, 1991) reflect either continued relevance or needed revisions. Additionally, the author recommends developmental stages from Bandura's *Social Learning Theory* in self-efficacy; Brofenbrenner's *Bioecological Theory* of roles, activities, and relationships; and Bruner's *Discovery Learning* in the role of developmental constructivism, to enhance the Llorens theory and schematic. This section concludes with a summary of these important considerations for the model's expansion.

Tracing the Model's History

To formulate a developmental theory for health and rehabilitation, Llorens (1970) drew her assumptions from the growth models presented by Ayres, Gesell, Erikson, Freud, Havighurst, Mosey, Pierce and Newton, and Piaget, and from her own professional experience and philosophy about the role of occupation in health and rehabilitation. Llorens presented her theoretical premises and constructs and then illustrated them in a three-part schematic model for practice as concurrent areas of growth and as temporal, chronological age levels. In Section 1, Llorens blends various theories in hierarchal and heuristic continuums of developmental expectations, behaviors, and needs that enable occupational performance. In Section 3, she presented the behavioral expectations and adaptive skills that one uses in the performance of occupational behavior roles related to environmental tasks, activities, and relationships. In Section 2, Llorens explained the role of purposeful activities (occupation) and relationships as occupational therapy's medium for practice in the adaptation process (Llorens, 1970).

Developmental Model's Thesis and Premises

Facilitating Growth and Development (Llorens, 1970; Walker & Shortridge, 1993) provides a theoretical model for occupational therapy to seek out, identify, and respond to a person's occupational performance needs. According to Mosey (1974), a theoretical model for practice "... provides certain assumptions, a theoretical base, and a set of operating principles" (p. 138). Llorens developed *Facilitating Growth and Development* from the following thesis:

> That occupational therapy is a facilitation process which assists the individual in achieving mastery of life tasks and the ability to cope as efficiently as possible with the life expectations made of him [or her] through the mechanisms of selected input stimuli and availability of practice in a suitable environment (Llorens, 1970, p. 93).

Llorens (1970) supported her thesis with the following premises:

1. That the human organism develops horizontally in the areas of neurophysiological, physical, psychosocial, and psychodynamic growth and in the development of social language, daily living, and sociocultural skills at specific periods of time;
2. That the human organism develops longitudinally in each of these areas in a continuous process as he ages;
3. That mastery of particular skills, abilities, and relationships in each of the areas of neurophysiological, physical, psychosocial, and psychodynamic development, social language, and daily living, and sociocultural skills, both horizontally and longitudinally, is necessary to the successful achievement of satisfactory coping behavior and adaptive relationships;
4. That such mastery is usually achieved naturally in the course of development;
5. That the fundamental endowment of the individual and the stimulation of experiences received within the environment of the family come together to interact in such a way as to promote positive early growth and development in both the horizontal and longitudinal planes;
6. That later the influences of extended family, community, social and civic groups assist in the growth process;
7. That physical or psychological trauma related to disease, injury, environmental insufficiencies, or intrapersonal vulnerability can interrupt the growth and development process;
8. That such growth interruption will cause a gap in the developmental cycle resulting in a disparity between expected coping behavior and adaptive facility and the necessary skills and abilities to achieve same;

9. That occupational therapy through the skilled application of activities [occupation] and relationships can provide growth and development links to assist in closing the gap between expectation and ability by increasing skills, abilities, and relationships in the neurophysiological, physical, psychosocial, psychodynamic, social language, daily living, and sociocultural spheres of development as indicated both horizontally and longitudinally.
10. That occupational therapy through the skilled application of activities [occupation] and relationships can provide growth experiences to prevent the development of potential maladaptation related to insufficient nurturance in neurophysiological, physical, psychosocial, psychodynamic, social language, daily living, and sociocultural spheres of development both horizontally and longitudinally (pp. 93–94).

Basic Concepts of Llorens' Schematic Model

Llorens' theoretical model (schematic) resulted from these constructs (thesis and supporting premises). According to Llorens, the human organism uses purposeful activities and relationships to adapt to developmental change in distinct phases and levels of growth throughout the life cycle. These changes occur through adaptive neurophysiological processing of internal and external stimuli in response to occupational demands that are activated by specific types of activities and affective object relationships and in accordance with the individual's dynamic genetic endowment and environmental context (Lorens, 1981a). The following definition of terms and discussion of Sections 1, 2, and 3 of Llorens' schematic refer to (a) the explanatory role of activities for occupational enablement and role acquisition (Section 1 and 3) and (b) the predictive role of occupational therapy in facilitating activities and relationships to accomplish same (Section 2) (see schematic in Figure 1).

Developmental Model Explained: Sections 1, 2, and 3 of Facilitating Growth and Development

Terminology

Definitions of terms in Table 1 that are used throughout Parts 1, 2, 3, and 4 of this book are provided after Figure 1.

FIGURE 1. Schematic Representation of Facilitating Growth and Development

Section 1
Developmental Expectations, Behaviors and Needs

Neurophysiological, Sensorimotor (Ayres)	Physical-Motor (Gesell)	Psychosocial (Erikson)	Psychodynamic (Grant/Freud)	Sociocultural (Gesell)	Social Language (Gesell)	Activity of Daily Living (Gesell)
0-2 yrs. Sensorimotor Tactile, vestibular, visual, auditory, olfactory, gustatory functions	0-2 yrs. Head sags Fisting Gross motion Walking Climbing	Basic Trust vs. Mistrust/Oral Sensory Ease of feeding Depth of sleep Relax. of bowels	0-4 yrs. Oral Dependency Init. aggress. Oral erotic activity	Individual mothering person most important Immediate family group important	Small sounds Coos Vocalizes Listens Speaks	Recognizes bottle Holds spoon Holds glass Controls bowel
6 mo.-4 yrs Integration of Body Sides Gross motor plan Form & space Balance Post. and bilateral integration Body scheme-develop.	2-3 yrs. Runs Balances Hand preference Coordination	Autonomy vs. Shame & Doubt/ Muscular-Anal Conflict between holding on & letting go	0-4 yrs. Independence Resistiveness Self-assertiveness Narcissism Ambivalence	Parallel play Often alone Recognizes extended family	Identifies objects verb. Asks "why?" Short sentences	Feeds self Helps undress Recognizes simple tunes No longer wets at night
3-7 Discrimination Refined tactile, kinesth, visual, auditory, olfact., gustatory functions	3-6 yrs. Coordination more graceful Muscles develop Skills develop	Initiative vs. Guilt/ Locomotor-Genital Aggressiveness Manipulation Coercion	3-6 yrs. Genital-Oedipal Genital interest Poss. of opp. parent Antag. to same parent Castration fears	Seeks companionship Makes decisions Plays with other children Takes turns	Combines talking and eating Complete sentences Imaginative Dramatic	Laces shoes Cuts with scissors Toilets independently Helps set table

3- Abstract Thinking Conceptualization Complex relations Read, write numbers	6-11 yrs. Energy development Skill practice to attain proficiency	Industry vs. Inferiority/Latency Wins recognition thru productivity Learns skills & tools	6-11 yrs. Latency Prim. struggles quiescent Init. in mastery of skills Strong defenses	Group play & team activities Independence of adults Gang interests	Enjoys dressing up Learns value of money Responsible for grooming
	11-13 yrs. Rapid growth Poor posture Awkwardness	Identity vs. Role Confusion/Puberty & Adolescence Identification Social Roles	11- Adolescence Emancip. from parents Occup. decisions Role experiment Re-exam of values	Team games Organization important Interest in opposite sex	Interest in earning money
		Intimacy vs. Isolation/Young Adulthood Commitments Body & ego mastery			
		Generativity vs. Stagnation/Adulthood Guiding next generation Creative, productive			
		Ego Integrity vs Despair/Maturity Acceptance of own life cycle			

Section 2
Facilitating Activities and Relationships (Selected)
Section 3
Behavior Expectations and Adaptive Skills

	Sensorimotor Activities	Developmental Play Activities	Symbolic Activities	Interpersonal Relationships	Developmental Tasks (Havighurst)	Ego-Adaptive Skills (Mosey, Pearce & Newton)
E V	Tactile Stim., Ident. Body parts, sounds, Objects	Dolls, Animals, Sand, Water, Excursions	Biting, Chewing, Eating, Blowing, Cuddling	Individual interaction	Learning to walk, talk, take solids, Elimination	Ability to respond to mothering, Mastering of gross motor responses
A L U	Phys. exercise, Balancing, Motor planning	Pull toys, Playground, Clay, Crayons, Chalk	Throwing, Dropping, Messing, Collecting, Destroying	Individual interaction, Parallel play	Sex difference, Form concepts of soc. & physical reality, Relate emotionally to others, Right vs. wrong, Develop a conscience	Ability to respond to routines of daily living, Mastery of 3 dimen. space, Sense of body image
A T I O N	Listening, Learning, Skilled tasks & games	Being read to, Coloring, Drawing, Painting	Destroying, Exhibiting	Individual interaction, Play small groups		Ability to respond to routines of daily living, Mastery of 3 dimen. space, Tolerate frustrations, Sit still, Delay gratification
	Reading, Writing, Numbers	Scooters, Wagons, Collections, Puppets, Building.	Controlling, Mastery	Individual interaction, Groups, Teams	Learn phys. skills, Getting along, Reading, writing, Values, Social attitudes	Ability to perceive, sort, organize & utilize stimuli, Work in groups, Master inanimate obj.

Weaving Machinery tasks Carving Modeling		More mature relationships Social roles Select occupation Achieving emot. independence	Ability to accept & discharge respn. Capacity for love
Arts Crafts Sports Club & interest groups Work	Individual interaction Groups	Selecting a mate Starting a family Marriage, home Congenial social group	Ability to function indep. Control drives Plan & execute Purposeful motions Obtain org. & use knowledge Part. in primary group Part. in variety of relationships Exp. self as accept. Part. in mutually satisfying heterosexual relations
		Civic & social responsibility Econ. standard of living Dev. adult leisure activities Adjust to aging parents Adjust to decr. phys. health, retire., death Age group affiliations Meeting social obligations	

From Llorens, L. A. (1970). Facilitating growth and development: The promise of occupational therapy. 1969 Eleanor Clarke Slagle Lecture. *American Journal of Occupational Therapy, 24*, 93-101. Section 1, p. 96 (Reproduced with Permission).

TABLE 1. Definition of Terms

Occupation (the state of being occupied)	An activity in which one engages (Merriam-Webster, 2005), as "a person's goal directed use of time, energy, interest, and attention" (Llorens, 1981b, p. 2).
Occupational association	The association of simultaneous and sequential stimuli (information) to select and/or retrieve and plan for object finding and using. Association used here connotes "the process of forming mental connections or bonds between sensations, ideas, or memories" (Merriam-Webster, 2005).
Occupational process	The use of occupational association for *doing- with meaning* (Fidler & Fidler, 1978) in purposeful object (animate and inanimate) action sequences (activity as means).
Occupational activity	The use of the occupational process to connect multiple body/mind components into a unified purposeful performance (ends) (Llorens, 1981a; Yerxa, 1994/1996).
Occupation form	The ecological objects/relationship used in the occupational activity (Nelson, 1986).
Vocation	"the work in which a person is regularly employed" (Merriam-Webster, 2005).
Occupational task	Represents a grouping of activities which have a similar productive role value (Llorens, 1991).
Occupational adaptation	A person's ecological adjustment to their occupational activity, task and role demands/expectations (Schultz & Schkade, 1992a, 1992b). Ecological means "the totality or pattern of relations between organisms and their environment" (Merriam-Webster, 2005).
Science of occupation (activity theory)	Purposeful engagement in activity (occupation) within relevant contexts. Incorporates multiple spheres of science; such as sociological theory, neurological theory, psychophysiological theory, developmental theory and occupational theory (Llorens, 1973, 1981a, 1981b, 1984a, 1984b, 1986, 1993; Llorens & Rubin, 1962; Humphry, 2005; West, 1984).
Activity components (enablers of occupation)	Neurophysiological, sensorimotor, physical, psychosocial, and psychodynamic growth; and social language, daily living, and sociocultural skills (Llorens, 1970, 1976).
Spatiotemporal adaptation	The neurophysiological process by which the distribution, timing, frequency, and amplitude of occupation enablers (as growth parameters) mature (Gilfoyle, Grady, & Moore, 1990). Distribution used in this sense means "the pattern of branching and termination of a ramifying structure (as a nerve)" (Merriam-Webster, 2005). Timing is used here to mean "to set the tempo, speed, or duration" (Merriam-Webster, 2005). Frequency is used to mean "the number of times that a periodic function repeats the same sequence of

(continued)

	values during a unit variation of the independent variable" (Merriam-Webster, 2005). By amplitude, it is meant the "extent or range of a quality, property, process, or phenomenon" (Merriam-Webster, 2005).
Central pattern generation	Rhythmical neurophysiological feed forward patterns, endogenously activated and sensorially mediated, for both occupational and spatiotemporal adaptation (Kuo, 2002; Marder & Bucher, 2001).
Occupational balance	The well-being that results from the synchronization of occupational associations with reality (Wilcock, 1999; Wright, 2004).
Occupational performance	The productive outcome of activities or tasks required by social and occupational role in the areas of work/education, leisure/play, self maintenance and rest (Baum & Law, 1997; Llorens, 1976).
Occupational performance enablers	The specific components of purposeful activity (see activity components) (Llorens, 1991).
Occupational performance roles	The occupational and social role behaviors connected with performance of occupational activities and tasks (Llorens, 1991)

Note: The definitions are presented as the terms relate to one another, rather than alphabetically.

Section 1. Developmental Expectations, Behaviors, and Needs

Llorens (1970) drew from activity theory and growth models (Llorens, 2004; Papalia et al., 2001) to construct a "loosely knit" developmental framework that describes phases and levels of developmental growth. People perform activities and engage in relationships that incorporate object-environmental reciprocity and that typify a specific developmental phase and role. In Section I, the activities and relationships typical of growth correlate to a person's intrapersonal and interpersonal environment of *neurophysiological, physical, psychosocial,* and *psychodynamic growth,* and development of *social language, daily living,* and *sociocultural* skills, all of which illustrate "Developmental Expectations, Behaviors, and Needs" (Llorens, 1970, p. 96 [Section 1 of the conceptual model]). Llorens illustrated these growth areas and relationships as activity component subskill areas that may categorically coexist within any given activity. An example of complimentary activity components *needed, expected,* and *behaviorally* observed is illustrated in playing baseball on a team during a baseball game. In this one integrated activity, a child needs good eye and hand coordination, physical strength, social-emotional stability, and regulation in intrapersonal and interpersonal relationships, motor skills, and planning language ideation to accompany the actions involved, the ability to tie her shoes (coordination) so that she doesn't trip and fall when she runs, and an environment suited to the activity. To provide an example of abilities needed in each of the activity component areas, Llorens identified behavioral and biologically based theorists who have contributed important explanations or observations of functioning within a specific component area. As noted in Figure 1, these areas include *neurophysiological, physical, psychosocial*, and *psychodynamic growth*, and development of *social language, daily living*, and *sociocultural* skills at specific growth periods in the developmental process.

Section 2. Facilitating Selected Developmental Activities and Relationships

According to occupational theory (Llorens, 1984a, 1984b), humans are fine tuned to recognize those activities and relationships that promote healthy growth, because activities and relationships contain intrinsic properties, which both internally and externally motivate, engage, and reinforce individual choice within a given developmental growth phase and context (Section 2 of the model pertaining to why occupational therapists use activities [occupation] and relationships). For example, during engagement in an breastfeeding activity where an infant is sucking at his mother's breast, multiple integrated activity components reinforce this activity. The infant receives internal nourishment, external warmth and tactile sensation, reciprocity and mutuality from mother/child interactions, opportunities for mastery of the suck-swallow-breathe pattern, efficient feeding coordination, and erotic sensations involving the oral erogenous zone. Hand in hand (co-occupationally), mother also receives occupational benefits from nursing, from multiple activity components that blend or integrate together as a complete activity. Llorens (1976) paraphrased the growth parameters of Section 1 activity components for *occupational performance* in activities and interpersonal relationships. These parameters, which reflect occupational enablement for occupation are sensorimotor efficiency and developmentally appropriate affective object relationships (Llorens, 1976). These qualitative abilities (composed of the sub-skill enablers from Section 1) undergird an individual's ability to adapt to developmental change and growth parameters, resulting in the occupational behaviors and adaptive skills found in Section 3. When examined together in continuums of function to dysfunction, these behaviors explain the need for the purposeful activities and relationships, detailed in Section 2 (see Figure 1).

Section 3. Developmental Behavior Expectations and Adaptive Skills

While Section 1 provides specific examples of important activity subskills illustrated by various growth models, Llorens uses Section 3 to portray how the activities and relationships in Section 1 are assimilated by people into larger tasks for roles that consist of similar kinds of occupational behaviors within daily routines. In a general sense, the activity of playing ball on a team during a ball game belongs in Section 3 as a developmental task of early childhood. Specific kinds of *developmental tasks* occur in specific contexts and relate to occupational behavior roles such as son, daughter, mother, worker, dancer, baseball player, and student. In turn, occupational task roles entail societal and personal expectations. Llorens (1970) postulated that occupational roles develop from the activity experiences of childhood enabled in the growth models of Section 1. As noted in Figure 1, Section 3, "Behavior Expectations and Adaptive Skills" (p. 97) consist of various *developmental tasks* and *ego-adaptive skills*. Just as specific activity components from Section 1 are illustrated as postulates regarding change in Section 2, one also finds in Section 2 the larger areas of occupational performance behaviors and skills needed for Section 3 as play/leisure, education/work, self-care, and rest/relaxation time activities. Occupational performance in the environmental context of role-bound behavior results from the enablement of growth, as efficient sensorimotor integration, and development of appropriate affective object relationships. In other words, Section 2 is utilized as a linkage between the two sections. It illustrates how an occupational therapist may use purposeful activities and relationships to intervene in deficits of *Developmental Expectations, Behaviors, and Needs* (Section 1) or *Behavior Expectations and Adaptive Skills* (Section 3).

Llorens' Subsequent Publications and Model Changes

Model Application and Conceptualization

Six years after publishing *Facilitating Growth and Development* ... , Llorens published *Application of a Developmental Theory for Health and Rehabilitation* (Llorens, 1976). She added more description to her schematic model to enhance its explanatory and predictive value, and applied her earlier (1970) theoretical formulations in a case study format with various ages and types of disabilities.

The various cases chosen by Llorens explained how a lack of mastery in the enabling sub-skill activities of Section 1 created maladaptation in the occupational tasks and roles for Sections 3. In particular, she noted how the cumulative effects of poorly integrated Section 1 activity components negatively impact the daily balance of performance in time usage for work/education, play/leisure crafts or games and sports, self-care (self-maintenance), and rest/relaxation occupations. These performance areas provide the medium for occupational therapists to interpret the occupational process and activities of Sections 1 and 3, and are used as postulates regarding change when problems in spatiotemporal or occupational adaptation occur in developmental expectations, behaviors, and needs (Section 1), or personal and social role expectations and ego adaptive skills (Section 3).

Although the above correlation of the relationship of Sections 1, 2, and 3 were conceptually expressed in writing in 1976 (p. 37) and 1984a and 1984b, it was not until Llorens wrote *Performance Tasks and Roles Throughout the Lifespan* (Llorens, 1991) that she illustrated her theoretical 1970 sections as a corollary concept; heuristic and hierarchal adaptive systems portrayed as levels of mastery in Figure 2.

Schematic Changes to the Developmental Theory 1976 and 1991

In her subsequent theoretical delineations, Llorens did not reformulate her theory in the sense of changing major constructs. Rather, she added more *depth* and *explanation* to demonstrate the continuity of each of the three sections (see Figure 3; the author italicized changes made by Llorens). For example, in Section 1, what began as "neurophysiological" in 1970 changed to

FIGURE 2. Heuristic and Hierarchal Adaptive Systems

Level 3	Occupational roles
	Worker, student, volunteer, homemaker, parent, son, daughter, mate, sibling, peer, and best friend/chum
Level 2	Activities and tasks of occupational performance
	Skill areas: Self-care/self-maintenance, play/leisure, work/education, and rest/relaxation
Level 1	Occupational performance enablers
	Subskills: Sensory perception, sensory integration, motor coordination, psychosocial and psychodynamic responses, sociocultural development, social language responses

From Llorens (1991). (Reproduced with Permission).

neuropsychological in 1991, while maintaining the sensorimotor (Ayres) emphasis in 1970, 1976, and 1991. This change reflected an ongoing trend in the *Sensory Integration Theory and Practice* (Bundy, Lane, & Murray, 2002) literature, where the typical development of sensorimotor integration results in the observation of neuropsychological outcomes, as Llorens indicated in the column heading change. In essence, the term *sensorimotor integration* means neurophysiological processing, so the change to neuropsychological avoided duplication and made this occupational component of *Developmental Expectations, Behaviors, and Needs* more succinct. Interestingly, she moved a psychodynamic behavior, oral erotic activity, to the sociocultural component area, perhaps to recognize the cultural expression of erogenous zone development. The other Section 1 additions to the various sub-skill component areas built upon already established processes and skills for behaviors seen in midlife and maturity.

In Section 2, *Facilitating Activities and Relationships (Selected)*, the changes in the *Sensorimotor Activities* column reflect the ongoing theory development in this activity component area; Llorens included more sensory systems. The addition of occupational performance outcome areas was of particular importance as Llorens added items to the *Developmental Play Activities* column, such as leisure time occupational activities, and terminology for education and work occupational performance time usage. With these changes, Llorens changed the column name in 1976 to *Developmental Activities*. Another important change in this section was the addition of the

FIGURE 3. Facilitation of Growth and Development (Llorens, 1991)

Section 1
Developmental Expectations, Behaviors and Needs

Neurophysiological, 1970, 1976 / *Neuropsychological, 1991* / Sensorimotor 1970, 1976, 1991 (Ayres)	Physical-Motor (1970, 1976, 1991) (Gesell)	Psychosocial (1970, 1976, 1991) (Erikson)	Psychodynamic (1970, 1976, 1991) (Grant/Freud)	Sociocultural (1970, 1976, 1991) (Gesell)	Social Language (1970, 1976, 1991) (Gesell)	Activity of Daily Living (1970, 1976, 1991) (Gesell)
0-2 yrs. Sensorimotor Tactile, vestibular, visual, auditory, olfactory, gustatory functions	0-2 yrs. Head sags Fisting Gross motion Walking Climbing	Basic Trust vs. Mistrust/Oral Sensory Ease of feeding Depth of sleep Relax. of bowels	0-4 yrs. Oral Dependency Init. aggress.	*Oral erotic activity; moved to this column from "Psychodynamic" in 1991* Individual mothering person most important Immediate family group important	Small sounds Coos Vocalizes Listens Speaks	Recognizes bottle Holds spoon Holds glass Controls bowel
6 mo.-4 yrs Integration of Body Sides Gross motor plan Form & space Balance Post. and bilateral integration Body scheme-develop.	2-3 yrs. Runs Balances Hand preference Coordination	Autonomy vs. Shame & Doubt/ Muscular-Anal Conflict between holding on & letting go	0-4 yrs. Independence Resistiveness Self-assertiveness Narcissism Ambivalence	Parallel play Often alone Recognizes extended family	Identifies objects verb. Asks "why?" Short sentences	Feeds self Helps undress Recognizes simple tunes No longer wets at night
3-7 yrs. Discrimination Refined tactile, kinesth, visual, auditory, olfact., gustatory functions	3-6 yrs. Coordination more graceful Muscles develop Skills develop	Initiative vs. Guilt/ Locomotor-Genital Aggressiveness Manipulation Coercion	3-6 yrs. Genital-Oedipal Genital interest Poss. of opp. parent Antag. to same parent Castration fears	Seeks companionship Makes decisions Plays with other children Takes turns	Combines talking and eating Complete sentences Imaginative Dramatic	Laces shoes Cuts with scissors Toilets independently Helps set table

3- yrs. Abstract Thinking, Conceptualization, Complex relations, Read, write numbers	6-11 yrs. Energy development, Skill practice to attain proficiency	Industry vs. Inferiority/ Latency, Wins recognition thru productivity, Learns skills & tools	6-11 yrs. Latency, Prim. struggles quiescent, Init. in mastery of skills, Strong defences	Group play & team activities, Independence of adults, Gang interests	*Added in 1976, continued in 1991*, *Language major form of communication*	Enjoys dressing up, Learns value of money, Responsible for grooming
Added in 1976, continued in 1991, *Continue to develop Conceptualization, Complex relations, Read, write numbers*	11-13 yrs. Rapid growth, Poor posture, Awkwardness	Identity vs. Role Confusion/Puberty & Adolescence, Identification, Social Roles	11- yrs. Adolescence, Emancip. from parents, Occup. decisions, Role experiment, Re-exam of values	Team games, Organization important, Interest in opposite sex	*Verbal language predominates*	Interest in earning money
Development presumably maintained	*Added in 1976, continued in 1991*, *Growth established and maintained*	Intimacy vs. Isolation/Young Adulthood, Commitments, Body & ego mastery	*Added in 1976, continued in 1991*, *Outgrow need for parent validation, Identify with others*	*Added in 1976, continued in 1991*, *Group affiliation, Family, social, civic interest*	Non-verbal behavior used	*Added in 1976, continued in 1991*
Alterations begin to occur in sensory functions, conceptualization, and memory	*Alterations begin to occur in motor behavior, strength, and endurance*	Generativity vs. Stagnation/Adulthood, Guiding next generation, Creative, productive	*Emotional responsibilities may lessen, Phys. and econ. independ. accepted, Shift from survival to enjoyment*			*Concern for personal grooming, mate, family* / *Accepting and adjusting to changes of middle age*
Alterations in sensory functions, conceptualization, and memory	*Alterations in motor behavior, strength and endurance*	Ego Integrity vs. Despair/Maturity, Acceptance of own life cycle	*Continued growth after middle age, Inner trend toward survival*			*Adjusting to changes after middle age*

Section 2
Facilitating Activities and Relationships (Selected)

Sensorimotor Activities (1970, 1976, 1991)	1970: Developmental Play Activities / 1976, 1991: Developmental Activities	Symbolic Activities (1970, 1976, 1991)	Daily Life Tasks (This section added in 1976, continued in 1991)	Interpersonal Relationships (1970, 1976) / Interpersonal Activities (1991)
1970: Tactlie Stim., Ident. Body parts, sounds, Objects *1976, 1991: Tactile, visual, aud., olfact., gust. Stimulation*	Dolls Animals Sand Water Excursions	Biting Chewing Eating Blowing Cuddling	*Recognize food* *Hold feeding equip.* *Use feeding equip.*	Individual interaction
Phys. Exercise Balancing Motor planning	Pull toys Playground Clay Crayons Chalk	Throwing Dropping Messing Collecting Destroying	*Feeding* *Toileting*	Individual interaction Parallel play

Listening Learning Skilled tasks & games	Being read to Coloring Drawing Painting	Destroying Exhibiting	*Feeding* *Dressing* *Toileting* *Simple chores*	Individual interaction Play Small groups
Reading Writing Numbers	Scooters Wagons Collections Puppets Bldg.	Controlling Mastery	*Feeding* *Dressing* *Grooming* *Spending*	Individual interaction Groups Teams Clubs
(Added 1976, continued, 1991) *All of the above available* *to be recycled*	Weaving Machinery tasks Carving Modeling	*(Added 1976, continued,* *1991)* *All of the above available* *to* *be recycled*	*Feeding* *Dressing* *Grooming* *Pre-voc. skills*	Individual interaction Groups Teams
	Arts Crafts Sports Club & interest groups Work		*Feeding* *Dressing* *Grooming* *Life role skills*	Individual interaction Groups
Education	*(Added 1976, continued,* *1991)*			

Section 3
Behavior Expectations and Adaptive Skills

Developmental Tasks (Havighurst)	Ego-Adaptive Skills (Mosey, Pearce & Newton)	Intellectual Development (This section added in 1976, continued in 1991) (Piaget)
Learning to walk, talk, take solids	Ability to respond to mothering	Motor skills
Elimination	Mastering of gross motor responses	Integrated
Sex difference		Investigative
Form concepts of soc. & physical reality	Ability to respond to routines of daily living	Imitative
Relate emotionally to others	Mastery of 3 dimen. space	Egocentric
Right vs. wrong	Sense of body image	
Develop a conscience		
	Ability to respond to routines of daily living	Egocentrism reduced, social increased,
	Mastery of 3 dimen. space	Lang. Rep. motor
	Tolerate frustrations	
	Sit still	
	Delay gratification	
Learn phys. skills	Ability to perceive, sort, organize & utilize stimuli	Orders experience
Getting along	Work in groups	Relates parts to wholes
Reading, writing	Master inanimate obj.	Deduction
Values		
Social attitudes		

22

More mature relationships Social roles Select occupation Achieving emot. independence	Ability to accept & discharge respn. Capacity for love	*Systematic approach to problems* *Sense of equality*
Selecting a mate Starting a family Marriage, home Congenial social group	Ability to function interpedently Control drives Plan & execute Purposeful motions Obtain org. & use knowledge Part. in primary group Part. in variety of relationships Exp. self as accept. Part. in mutually satisfying heterosexual relations	*Development established and maintained*

Civic & social responsibility
Econ. standard of living
Dev. adult leisure activities
Adjust to aging parents
  Adjust to decr. phys. health, retire.,
  death
Age group affiliations
  Meeting social obligations
		Alterations in other areas may affect

From Llorens, L. A. (1991). Performance tasks and roles throughout the lifespan. In C. Christiansen & C. Baum (Eds.), *Occupational therapy: Overcoming human performance deficits* (pp. 45-66). Thorofare, NJ: Charles B. Slack, p. 48-49. (Reproduced with Permission).

entire column of *Daily Life Tasks*, which Llorens conceptualized as
concerned with survival serving (food, shelter, warmth, elimination)
versus play-based activities, and resulting in Life Role (occupational
performance) Skills (Llorens, 1981a). Last, Llorens changed the column *Interpersonal Relationships* in 1991 to *Interpersonal Activities*,
presumably to maintain the emphasis of this section as purposeful
activity.

In Section 3, Llorens added Piaget. Initially, intellectual functions had been addressed under sensorimotor activities in Section
1. However, adding Piaget to the *Behavior Expectations and Adaptive Skills*, Section 3 recognizes the larger role of cognition in the
adaptive expression of *Developmental Tasks* and *Ego Adaptive
Skills*, which all together support occupational and social role
behaviors.

Activity Theory, Growth Models, and the Change Process: Developmental Theorists Represented by Llorens

Mapping New Directions

Llorens' vision for *Facilitating Growth and Development* (Llorens,
1970) incorporated multiple theorists. She chose the theorists from
the biological and behavioral sciences to provide growth models
pertaining to the "sociocultural environment and the biological-
psychological environment" (Llorens, 1984a, p. 30). These models
are operationalized by occupational science (activity) theory to
explain how activity components are interwoven throughout development as a determinant of change. To promote this integration, occupational therapy intervention (Section 2) uses interpersonal
relationships and occupational readiness activities for occupational
enablement of internal neurophysiological spatiotemporal adaptation
and occupational activities and interpersonal relationships for the
external occupational adaptation processes.

Purposeful activity and relationships occurring "in an environment
suitable for practice" (Llorens, 1970, p. 93), provide the context for
occupational therapy intervention. Environment refers to the ecology
of an individual's multiple adaptive systems, with the individual
representing the first level of the environment (Llorens, 1984a). This
idea is expressed in premises 3, 5, and 6 (Llorens, 1970), "... to permit
understanding [of] the person-environment and the application of

purposeful activity or occupation to bring about change in the occupational performance [activity] components, [areas of] occupational performance, and occupational [role] behavior of the client" (Llorens, 1984a, p. 33). Llorens illustrated this concept in Figure 2.

Llorens' use of activity theory and growth models to formulate the thesis, premises, and schematic model for her theory quite probably influenced the basic tenants and philosophy of the occupational therapy profession (American Occupational Therapy Association [AOTA], 1979). This philosophy states:

> Man [humankind] is an active being whose development is influenced by the use of purposeful activity. Using their capacity for intrinsic motivation, human being[s] are able to influence their physical and mental health and their social and physical environment through purposeful activity. Human life includes a process of continuous adaptation. Adaptation is a change in function that promotes survival and self-actualization. Biological, psychological, and environmental factors may interrupt the adaptation process at any time throughout the life cycle. Dysfunction may occur when adaptation is impaired. Purposeful activity facilitates the adaptive process.
>
> Occupational therapy is based on the belief that purposeful activity (occupation), including its interpersonal and environmental components, may be used to prevent and mediate dysfunction and to elicit maximum adaptation. Activity as used by the occupational therapist includes both an intrinsic and a therapeutic purpose (p. 785).

Coping with life's expectations through mastery of occupational tasks and the development of ego adaptive skills enlists the basic biological and behavioral components of activity (premise 3), linked by *occupational associations* and *process* to activate the internal and external motivation, affect, and object relationships inherent and autonomous to the activity. Adolf Meyer (1921/1996), a psychiatrist and proponent of occupation therapy, proposed that occupations "... expand into laws of growth and laws of function ... to fulfill the lifecycle of the human individual happily and effectively. ..." (p. 30). *Occupations* or *purposeful activities*, performed as a balanced and personally gratifying use of time, promote growth and development throughout the lifespan because of meaningful engagement.

Philosophically, occupations provide an *organizing (integrating)*
medium for humankind's deficits in environmental *adaptation*
(AOTA, 1979; Meyer, 1921/1996, Llorens, 1970, 1976, 1984a,
1984b, 1991).

Llorens conceptualized activity theory as a theory of occupation
science, standing side by side biological and behavioral science theories, as shown in Figure 4 (Llorens, 1984b). She linked occupational
theory to Section 2 of her theory regarding the prescriptive value of
purposeful activity and the application of relationships as adminis-
tered by occupational therapists. She also asserted that occupational
theory and the science of occupation must be verified to discern the
intrinsic and extrinsic value of purposeful activities or occupation
and relationships to elicit an adaptive behavioral response. Llorens
(1984b) noted that "in 1960, Jane Ayres had identified the value of
purposeful activities [as] the link that unites occupational therapy
for emotional as well as physical conditions" (p. 5). The relationship
between the theorists that Llorens drew from for her theory is parallel
to the relationship between the biological and behavioral sciences
(Sections 1 and 3) and occupational theory (Section 2). This relationship is noted in Figure 4.

An Examination of the Theorists Cited by Llorens

The author reviewed the theorists Llorens used in the schematic model, including those added to her schematic model in 1976
and 1991. This review was undertaken in two ways. First, the theorists' ideas were reviewed through the primary sources. These sources
were as follows: Ayres (1972, 1974), Erikson (1964), Freud (1938),
Gesell and Ilg (1949), Grant (1963), Hall (1954), Havighurst (1972),
Llorens and Rubin (1967), Mosey (1974, 1986, 1992), Pearce and
Newton (1963), Peck and Havighurst (1960), Piaget (1952).

Second, secondary sources were reviewed as follows: Ayres (Bundy
et al., 2002; Fisher, Murry, & Bundy, 1991), Erikson (Coles, 2000),
Freud (Breger, 2000; Grant, 1963; Schellenburg, 1978), Gesell
(Sroufe, Cooper, & DeHart, 1996), Grant (1963) derived a typology
of various emotional disorders based upon Freud, and Piaget
(Kegan, 1982). Additional authors who provided an overview of
current developmental theories and reviewed one or more of these
theorists were Case-Smith (2005), Cronin and Mandich (2005), Maier
(1978), Papalia et al. (2001), and Sroufe et al. (1996).

FIGURE 4. Theoretical Basis Common to Occupational Therapy

Sociological Theory Relating to	Neurological Theory Relating to	Psychophysiological Theory Relating to	Developmental Theory Relating to	Occupational Theory Relating to
Cultural value systems, role of activity, language, customs, and environment	Nervous system as the organizer/integrator of sensory stimuli	Mind/body mediated and integrated through the nervous system and manifested in behavior	Hierarchical, sequential, and simultaneous growth occurring through the lifespan	Inherent qualities of occupation (purposeful activity eliciting intrinsic motivation and extrinsic reinforcement for change and adaptation)

From Llorens (1984b). (Reproduced with Permission).

Impression of Theorists' Continued Relevance to the Llorens Model

All of the theorists Llorens drew from to formulate the behavioral and biological aspects of her theory remain relevant, except for needed changes to Freud as noted in Breger (2000), Papalia et al. (2001), and Schellenburg (1978). The author makes recommendations for changes to the psychodynamic aspect of Llorens' model in the next section.

Additionally, specific aspects of Peck, Kohlberg, and Maslow's theories were either mentioned in the Llorens 1991 text (Llorens, 1991) or added to her schematic model. Specifically, she noted Peck's work in the area of socially determined ego adaptive skills in adult development (p. 53), and these ideas were added to her model (in 1991) to expand Erikson's psychosocial stages of growth and development in maturity. Although Llorens noted Kohlberg's cognitive expansion of Piaget's concept of morality in her text (p. 53), these ideas were correlative in nature and were therefore not added to her schematic model. Llorens (1991) also cited Abraham Maslow's *Hierarchy of Needs* (p. 52). As with Kohlberg, Maslow's theory was intended to compliment the theme of mastery in the developmental process.

Suggested Modifications to the Psychodynamic Schematic Component

Needed Changes

As noted under *Impression of Theorists Continued Relevance ...,* the author's review of more recent literature based upon the writings of Freud indicate a need for some substantial changes in Llorens' schematic model in the area of psychodynamics. The rationale for change is as follows.

In her theoretical conceptualization of psychodynamics, Llorens based her schematic formulation upon the writings of Hall (1954), Grant (1963), and in her 1991 manuscript, Papalia and Olds (1986). While the genius of Freud is undisputed (Breger, 2000), more recent publications challenge Freud's assertions regarding the underlying psychosexual motives that he attributed to the *oedipus complex*, in particular the concepts of the castration complex, penis envy, and sexual orientation identification (Papilla et al., 2001; also see Breger, 2000; Kegan, 1982), which have not been verified. However, research has validated (to varying degrees) the oral and anal stage personality types and emergent feelings of conflict toward the same sex parent during the oedipal complex (Breger, 2000; Kegan, 1982; Papilia et al., 2001; Peck & Havighurst, 1960).

Evaluation and Recommended Revisions to Freud's Psychosexual Stages

The author reviewed various sources pertaining to Freud's writings, personal life, and letters (Breger, 2000), and Freud's account of *Infant and Child Sexuality* (Freud, 1938). This account was compared to Llorens' conceptualization. Three discoveries were made that provided a new perspective to the explanatory value of the topic of psychodynamics to occupation.

First, Sigmund Freud's work characterized the development of psychic processes in relationship to the gratification of erotic instincts (Freud, 1938; Hall, 1954; Winkelmann, 1959). His theoretical formulations proposed that erotic-based impulses form the foundation for socially expressed object choices and identifications. These object choices provide the emotional basis for occupational associations, process, and performance. The author decided to expand the psychodynamic component of Llorens' schematic to indicate the relationship between erogenous zone object choice and affective development.

> Sensuality is usually discussed in terms of the central appreciation of those complex stimuli and associations that give rise to it. Much of the primary erotic stimulus comes from the skin, and a definition in terms of the sensory receptors of the skin should be a necessary part of our understanding of the physical part of this complex sensation. It is hoped that those who study human behavior will find [this] ... anatomic and developmental information useful (Winkelmann, 1959, first para.).

Freud speculated that the developmental arousal of erogenous zones occurs through a mechanism in the central nervous system called central pattern generation "which is projected into the peripheral erogenous zone" (Freud, 1938, p. 588). (More detail and

description will be given to the central pattern generation concept in
Part 3 of this book.) In his chapters on *Infant Sexuality* and *The
Transformations of Puberty*, Freud asserted that sexual excitement
in the erotic zone areas stimulate an urge for gratification. Object-
action sequences directed to satisfy the "tickle" sensations result in
pregenital masturbatic activities of all zones. This means that centrally generated impulses stimulate oral, anal, genital, and visual
zones with an urge toward tension reduction. Objectifying these zones
enhances tactile localization, attention, and identification of tickle
areas, in turn promoting kinesthetic awareness, object finding, and
a desire for repetition of stimulation to the zone area.

The concept of centrally generated patterned impulses that inspire
directed activity sequences through object selection that is reinforced by zone area tissue, richly endowed for sensory reception,
is very different from a general maturation perspective of passive
zone sensitivity (without the central pattern generator perspective).
In other words, arousal of erogenous zone tissues (oral, genital,
anal, etc.) stem from centrally projected impulses "which... [are]
projected into the peripheral erogenous zone" (Freud, 1938, p.
588), thereby stimulating a yearning for gratification. Quite possibly, Freud's background in physiology may have led him to
hypothesize that central pattern generation directly influences
erogenous zone activity. Also, von Holst (1973), an early central
pattern generator theorist and neurophysiologist, may have influenced Freud as a contemporary.

The author also found a theme running through Freud's discussion of infantile sexuality as an autoerotic activity of genital
area masturbation. Freud divided genital masturbation into three
different age ranges, but acknowledged that it may run throughout
the pregenial period without interruption, including during
"latency." Interestingly, Llorens (versus Papalia et al., 2001, or
others) referred to infant and child masturbation as *narcissism* in
her schematic, but only in the initial infant period of 0–4 years.
The fact that masturbation is still a taboo to discuss raises some
interesting questions.

Cornog (2004) cited Freud on the inexhaustibility of the subject of
masturbation. However, she noted that, of the 30 books written since
the 1960s about masturbation, seven of these books are not considered literary works. Then, only 13 books were published since
the 1990s, and five since 2000, even though masturbation is

considered "the second most common sex act" (p. 310). She cited Bockting and Coleman's (2003) book, which includes five sections pertaining to recently published research on the topic of masturbation: women reporting its use early in childhood, the relationship between masturbation and intercourse, the inference that interest in intercourse does not decrease with the occurrence of masturbation, and, finally, Coleman's essay describing "the links between masturbation, sexual development, and adjustment...[and] the needs for future research" (p. 311). Cornog's review supports Freud's contentions regarding masturbation as a natural phenomena of childhood.

Finally, personality development is related to erogenous zone development in the developmental aspects of psychosexual stage development. In turn, personality is viewed as an outward manifestation of character development. "In a very real sense, assessing moral character is simply one way of assessing an individual's personality" (Peck & Havighurst, 1960, p. 11). In fact, Peck and Havighurst (1960) developed a motivational theory for developmental levels of character development that significantly correlate to six personality characteristics, all relevant to moral character development: (a) moral stability, (b) ego strength, (c) superego strength, (d) spontaneity, (e) friendliness, and a (f) hostility-guilt complex (p. 21). They cite Fenichel, who was paraphrasing Freud:

> Character [is] the habitual mode of bringing into harmony the tasks presented by internal demands and by the external world...[It] is necessarily a function of the constant, organized, and integrating part of the personality which is the ego.... The latest complication in the structure of the ego, the erection of the superego, is also decisive in forming the habitudinal patterns of character. What an individual considers good or bad is characteristic for him; likewise, whether or not he takes the commands of his conscience seriously, and whether he obeys his conscience or tries to rebel against it (Peck & Havighurst, 1960, pp. 1–2).

Hall (1954) noted that the pregenital phases (oral, anal, and phallic) with their associated object cathexes (both intra- and interpersonally in regard to sucking, expelling, or retaining feces, and masturbation), fuse with the genital phase object choices "to become a part of the permanent character structure" (p. 113). Last, the significance between personality and erogenous zone development is characterized by Hall in the following manner:

> The erogenous zones are of great importance for the development of personality because they are the first important sources of irritating excitations which the baby has to contend and they yield the first important experiences of pleasure. Moreover, actions involving the erogenous zones bring the child into conflict with his parents, and the resulting frustrations and anxieties stimulate the development of a large number of adaptations, displacements, defenses, transformations, compromises, and sublimations (Hall, 1954, p. 103).

Summary of recommended psychosexual revisions. In summary, Freud's conception of centrally generated impulses that stimulate erogenous zone development should be included in the psychodynamics section. The psychosexual developmental phases should also include affective object cathexes/choice. The inclusion of these zones and their object choices is important because all zones are active and sensorially integrative with the primary zone for each developmental phase during growth and development. The integrative mechanism for psychosexual object relations occurs through occupational associations, process, and performance. Consequently, the author suggests a modification of Llorens' psychodynamic component; that is, to split (divide) the psychodynamic section into two parts to illustrate the revision in Freud's psychosexual developmental phases and a new section created for character development. The following discussion highlights the important research findings of Peck and Havighurst (1960), impressively carried out as a mixed method study on the developmental phases of moral character development.

Moral Character Development: A Proposed Addition to Psychodynamics

Peck and Havighurst (1960) developed a motivational theory for moral character, with *moral* defined as a person's motivation and intent "to do good or ill to other people" (p. 2). While these stages were "each conceived as representative of a successive stage in the psychosocial development of the individual" (p. 3), they can also be used as a typology for character analysis (as correlates to Freud's psychosexual stages, Piaget's formulations of moral development [p. 19], and Fromm's formulation of ethical developmental stages [p. 3]). The following topology is based upon the *Maturity of Character Scale* (pp. 3–11; see definitions on Table 2, and model on Table 3):

1. Infancy: The *amoral* character "follows whims and impulses . . . to direct self-gratification" (p. 5) to the exclusion of social adaptation, and therefore lacks "internalized moral principals, conscious, or superego" (p. 5). This type of character may even seem attractive, much like an infant. Social mal-adaptation resulting in harmful behavior may be unintentional.
2. Early Childhood: The *expedient* character conforms socially to present an image of morality for appearances, which is easily abandoned for personal "want and needs" (p. 5). Superficial concern for others' well being is cast aside, especially when dishonesty can go unnoticed. Although ego skills may be intact, the conscience and superego are not consistently rational.
3. Later Childhood: Either (one of) the *conforming* or *irrational-conscientious* character types are symbolic of this period of growth. They are both representative of "fixation at the later pregenital stages, extending through the latency period" (p. 10).
   a. *Conforming* character follows prescribed social rules of conduct, regardless of their effect Personal gain may be ignored if the behavior constitutes a "departure from the prescribed rules of conduct" (p. 7), even if these rules are inconsistent or hateful for different persons or groups. A "crude conscience" (p. 7) is indicated by the rule bound behavior; however, morality of consequences do not determine behavior.
   b. *Irrational-conscientious* character follow a set of rigid internalized ideals, regardless of social mores or the effect of such actions on others. "This is the 'blind' rigid superego at work" (p. 7). Parent's values are inherited, which may "be reasonably effective in insuring outwardly moral behavior at all times" (p. 8).
4. Adolescence to adulthood: *Rational-altruistic* character type represents a morally mature and stable individual who uses rational judgment (both consciously and unconsciously) to guide interpersonal activities. This qualitative aspect of reasoning is based upon emotional stability and enables objectivity in decision making. Productive work includes motivation to act for the

TABLE 2. Definition of Terms of Table 3 on Psychodynamic Development

Erotism and autoerotism	In erotism, the child directs the impulse for gratification toward an outside course, such as the breast for nursing. Freud (1938) borrows the term "autoerotic" from Ellis to mean "the child [person] gratifies himself on his own body" (p. 586). He also explains that the urge to do so is initiated from within.
Centrally generated impulses	Central pattern generation arises intrinsically from various locations within the CNS as nerve (energy) impulses creating activity sequences that are genetically activated (endogenous) and exogenously (activities that are external) reinforced.
Erogenous zones	1. "It is a portion of skin or mucus membrane in which stimuli produce a feeling of pleasure of definite quality" (Freud, 1938, p. 587). 2. a. Nonspecific: sensitive areas on the body, such as the axillas, back of the neck, and sides of the thorax. b. Specific, acute erotic perception: "genital regions, including the prepuce, penis, clitoris, and external vulva of the female and perianal skin, lip, nipple, and conjunctiva [of the eye] as mucocutaneous end organs . . . (Winkelmann, 1959, p. 39). In addition to the prolific nerve endings in each of these zones, the hand is also equipped to sensorially appreciate input in tactile zones. "Compared with lower animals, the primate group is much better equipped to appreciate sensations in special tactile zones (Winkelmann, 1959).
Object-finding	Searching for and locating an object, animate or inanimate, to make an emotional investment in.
Occupational association	The ability to isolate and correlate simultaneous stimuli, sequentially, to plan and adapt for engagement by object finding and using. In regard to erogenous zone maturation and occupational association, "The pleasant associations and the learned and anticipated responses concurrent with the stimulus produce the final amplified central sensation" (Winkelmann, 1959, 2nd para.).
Occupational engagement	Participation in intrapersonal and interpersonal affective object relationships
Object choice/cathexes	"The investment of energy in the image of an object or the expenditure of energy in discharge action upon an object that will satisfy an instinct" (Hall, 1954, p. 39).
Object identification	"When the idea of the object agrees with the object itself, the idea is said to be identified with the object" (Hall, 1954, p. 42).

common good of others as much as for one's self. This typology is not meant to address the intricacies of the experimental or exploratory character of adolescence. The reader may use any number of theoretical frameworks along with the moral character types described in Table 3.

Summary of moral character addition to psychodynamics. In summary, Peck and Havighurst (1960) developed a theory of moral character development, with sequences and corresponding age phases. However, the authors' stress that this scale is approximate in nature and also that most adult personalities, at various times during the growth and development process, consist of a mixture of these characteristics. Last, the authors equate their developmental levels of moral character to Freud's psychosexual stages. They noted that the amoral type is posited to reflect character development in the oral stage; the expedient type is posited to reflect character development in the beginning stages of the anal phase of development; the character types of conformist and irrational-consciousness are posited to reflect a fixated character development in the pregenital phases extending through latency. And last, but not least, the emergence and synthesis of the rational-altruistic type is hypothesized to reflect growth beginning at the genital phase, as a life-long endeavor (Peck & Havighurst, 1960). Other frameworks, such as described by Glovinsky (2005), could be suitably used with this typology.

Linking Psychosexual and Character Development Together

Moral character development is posited to reflect the outward manifestation of a person's dynamic personality, as influenced through psychosexual development (see Tables 2 and 3). Table 2 describes pertinent terms specifically related to the topic of psychosexual erogenous zone development and to the psychological aspect of moral character development through occupation. The author's objective on Table 3 is to further define psychosexual development, to describe the affective objective relations and emotional significance of erogenous zone development, and to link psychosexual and moral character together through psychodynamics. The author posits this linkage through erogenous zone object-action sequences as an iterative process.

TABLE 3. Comparison of Stages of Psychodynamic Growth and Development of Freud with Peck and Havighurst

Psychodynamic Growth and Development			Character (habitual patterns represented by daily tasks) (Peck & Havighurst, 1960) — Impact of Peer and Family Relationships (Interpersonal Relationships)
Psychosexual Development (conscious and unconscious)	Occupational Association and Engagement (Affective Object Relations)	General Emotional Significance of Erogenous Zone Development	Levels of (Moral) Character Maturity (character development)
Libidinal Energy (centrally generated impulses) for Intrapersonal and Object Relation (interpersonal relationships involving people, places, and concepts) activities (Freud, 1938). Development through Erogenous Zone maturation			
S. Freud, (1938) Infantile – Puberty Sexuality Erogenous zone tissues and intrapersonal psychosexual development.	S. Freud, (1938) Erogenous zone tissues and interpersonal object relations (object choice/ cathexes/identification)	S. Freud (1938)	R. Peck and R. Havighurst (1960)
Infant Activity: 0-18 months (autoerotic) a. Lips: sucking primary activity; nutritive/ non-nutritive b. Genital masturbation (centrally determined tickling sensation demanding gratification) by "a rubbing contiguity with the hand'" (p. 590) in boys, and a "pressure reflex" (p. 590) by closing thighs (girls). c. Anal zone awareness; ambivalence d. Eyes: Visual exploration, "looking" e. Hands: Similar tissue sensitivity	Infant 0-3 years Lip tissue: Objects are breast, thumb, pacifier Anal and genital tissue stimulation: Object (person) relationships reinforce (unintentional) zone arousal during caretaking (bathing, cleaning and dressing), holding, rocking, and play Eyes and Hands: looking, touching, and manipulating	a. Regulation of homeostasis through nourishment, sleep induction, relaxation, elimination b. Pleasure of sexual feeling "of a definite quality" (p. 587) awakens desire for repetition, "...and may be able to influence the availability of voluntary attention" (p. 603). c. Foundation for later primacy, roles, personality stability d. "Primacy in the service of reproduction" (p. 598). e. "Stimulate the development of a large number of adaptations, displacements, defenses, transformations, compromises, and sublimations" (Hall, 1954, p. 103)	Infancy: The *Amoral* character "follows whims and impulses....to direct self gratification" (p.5) to the exclusion of social adaptation, and therefore lacks "internalized moral principles, conscious, or superego" (p. 5). This type of character may even seem attractive, much like an infant. Social mal-adaptation resulting in harmful behavior may be unintentional.
Child Activity: 18 months-3 years a. Lips: nutritive/ non-nutritive b. genital masturbation is cyclic and oscillating, interspersed with latency. c. Anal-sadistic phase: initial awareness leads to pleasurable holding back (masturbatic control) of fecal masses. Autoerotism increases with control. d. Eyes: visual exploration, "looking" discrimination.	Additional: sensory activities which enhance bodily arousal (all ages) also increase erogenous zone awareness. Likewise, erogenous arousal creates bodily arousal in other sensory and bodily systems.		

TABLE 3. Continued

Child Activity: 3-6 years a. Lips: nutritive/ non-nutritive b. Genital masturbation is manifested in the 3rd and 4th years. c. Anal: continued awareness and sphincter (active/passive) coordination d. Eyes: visual exploration, "looking" at playmates and adult genitalia, and observing toileting, increases. Interest in knowledge acquisition increases.	Child 3-6 years Phallic Period: Social experience (object relationships) pivotal in character development. Strong object investment (love object), deep affection for opposite sex parent, and gender identification (authority struggle) same sex parent. Knowledge sublimation for investigative activities.	Early Childhood: The *Expedient* character conforms socially to present an image of morality for appearances, which is easily abandoned for personal "want and needs" (p.5). Superficial concern for others well being is cast aside especially when dishonesty can go unnoticed. Although ego skills may be intact, the conscience and superego are not consistently rational.
Child Activity: 6-12 years a. Lips: nutritive/ non-nutritive b. Genital masturbation may be suppressed (through "moral defense forces" (p. 584) such as "loathing, shame and moral and esthetic ideal demands" (p. 583), "or it may continue without interruption" (591). c. Anal: continued muscular control and sphincter (active/passive) coordination d. Eyes: object attractors, knowledge and investigation, continued.	Child 6-12 years Latent or Partial Latency due to sexual inhibition; however "the influx of...sexuality does not stop even in this latency period..." (P. 584) For autoerotism (footnote, p. 591).	Later Childhood: Either character types are symbolic of this period of growth. *Conforming* character follows prescribed social rules of conduct, even if these rules are inconsistent or hateful for different persons or groups. A "crude conscience" (p. 7) is indicated by the rule bound behavior, however morality of consequences do not determine behavior. *Irrational-Conscientious* character follow a set of rigid internalized ideals, regardless of social mores or the effect of such actions on others. "This is the 'blind,' rigid superego at work" (p. 7).
Puberty to Adulthood a. Lips: kissing b. Genital Maturation: Ability for primacy for the purpose of procreation. c. Anal: continued muscular control and sphincter (active/passive) coordination Breasts: (women) maturation as erogenous zone and attractor. d. Eyes: Visual excitement of sexual objects (images, symbols)	Puberty to adulthood Independence from parents, selection of love object, sexual aims for tension reduction, sublimation of sexual energy for creativity. Ability to love, to produce.	Adolescence and Adulthood: *Rational-Altruistic* character type represents a morally mature and stable individual who uses rational judgment (both consciously and unconsciously) to guide interpersonal activities. This qualitative aspect of reasoning is based upon emotional stability, and enables objectivity in decision making. Productive work includes motivation to act for the common good of others as much as for one's self.

Conclusion: Recommended Modification to Psychodynamics

In summary, the author suggests that psychosexual object action sequences are linked to erogenous zone development. Peck and Havighurst (1960) posited that moral character development is a reflection of personality. These psychosexual stages, as proposed by Freud, occur through oscillating discharges of rhythmical central nervous system pattern generation for each zone. Hence, the author speculates that central pattern generation, in association with occupation in the socio-cultural milieu, is a causal factor in the development of personal psychodynamics. According to Llorens (1970) psychodynamics, as a component of occupational activity theory, plays a major role in the contribution to behavior and to socio-cultural norms. The author applies the psychosexual and character developmental phases, listed in Table 3 in Part 3 of this issue, as a modification to Llorens' schematic of psychodynamics. Next, the author reviews three new theorists, whose work has thus far not been discussed or included in the Llorens model.

Analysis of Three New Theorists for the Expansion of Facilitating Growth and Development in Occupational Therapy

This section presents the work of three new theorists who have thus far not been discussed. Indeed, their contributions to the discipline of psychology and to the educational and health care systems are immense. Albert Bandura's well-known performance-based model of self-efficacy is derived from social learning theory (Bandura, 1977a). Bandura has described the role of self-regulation through observational learning and the establishment of antecedent behaviors as related to cognition (Bandura, 1977a), behavior change and health promotion (Bandura, 1977b, 2004), development across the life span (Bandura, 1994), affective psychosocial functioning (Bandura, Caprara, Barbaranelli, Gerbino, & Pastorelli, 2003), and by others, in parenting high-risk infants (Hess, Teti, & Hussey-Gardner, 2004). Two other well-know and distinguished psychologists, Urie Bronfenbrenner and Jerome Brunner, were co-founders of Head Start (see Ziegler and Valentine, 1979) (Bruner, 1999). Additionally, both Bronfenbrenner and Bruner have made individual contributions to developmental constructivist theory, with Bronfenbrenner's evolving *Bioecological Theory and Model* (Brofenenbrenner, 1975, 1977, 1979, 2000; Bronfenbrenner & Ceci, 1994) and Bruner's theory of *Discovery*

Learning in development (Bruner, 1975), education (Bruner, 1966), and play (Bruner, 1976). The author describes these three theorists' major ideas in the following paragraphs and provides a *developmental phase sequence* for each.

Proposed Addition of Albert Bandura to Llorens' Theory: Performance-Based Treatment Strategies

The thesis of Bandura's work centers on the social-cognitive aspects through which learning occurs. An outshoot of learning theory or behaviorism (Papalia et al., 2001), *Social Learning Theory*, capitalizes upon the cognitive aspects of awareness, attention, retention, motivation, and enculturation. Although Bandura (1977a) acknowledges the role of genetics in behavior, he posited that behavioral change would not be possible if the social aspects of learning did not supply the relevancy of the task context, as a type of *psychic determinism*, versus pure biological *determinism*, or *behaviorism* (Bandura, 1977a). "Within this approach, symbolic, vicarious, and self-regulatory processes assume a prominent role" (p. 12). Bandura noted that people learn through observation and performance of social modeling. By observing others actions, and their consequences, humans "acquire large, integrated patterns of behavior without having to form them gradually by trial and error" (p. 12). Above all else, social learning theory assigns a "... prominent role to self-regulatory capacities" (p. 13).

To capture the role of self-regulatory capacities in daily tasks, Bandura (1977b) presented his theory of self-efficacy in the context of social cognitive learning experience. For Bandura, coping with life's expectations means developing the cognitive schematics in which linguistic and visual symbols and images are encoded in memory for retrieval in the performance of daily life occupations. The cognitive change process through which self-efficacy occurs ultimately functions as a regulatory adaptive mechanism to prepare people for judgment of their ability to function within a given context.

Through past performance, vicarious observational learning, verbal (extortive) persuasion, and emotive (physiologically arousing) external stimuli, a person's expectations about their experiences are motivationally imbued with meaning about their self-efficacy as a source of self-empowerment in occupational activities, tasks, and relationships. Individuals analyze expectations in regard to their strength and magnitude by assessing perceived capability to make an impact in various contexts. "Given appropriate skills and adequate incentives, however, efficacy expectations are a major determinant of people's choices of activities, how much effort they will expend, and how long they will sustain effort in dealing with stressful situations..." (Bandura, 1977b, p. 194). Interestingly, Bandura uses activities relevant to occupational therapy as the occupational means to achieve self-efficacy. He noted "...performance-based treatments not only promote behavioral accomplishments but also extinguish fear arousal" (p. 195). He noted also that people are able to generalize their performance when their feelings of efficacy are high, versus "... preoccupation with personal inadequacies" (p. 195).

Development and exercise of self-efficacy over the lifespan (Bandera, 1994, 4th para.). Bandura noted that "different periods of life present certain competency demands for successful functioning" (Bandura, 1994, 1st para.). These relative stages do not represent precisely determined levels of self-efficacy acquisition. Rather, these lifespan periods highlight the development of self-efficacy ability.

1. Infancy: Children learn from what they observe about their own actions. Their sense of self-efficacy is shaped by their perceived performance and its social and environmental impacts. Observations of one's own actions compared to other's actions leads to differentiation of self from others. Successful results in obtaining desired objects leads to an enhanced (competent) symbolic representation of the self.
2. Childhood: Family (parents, siblings), peers, and schools provide a context for judging personal efficacy. Peers exert a major influence through positive and/or negative feedback. Growth and development of self-efficacy can be facilitated or retarded. Perceived social efficacy can lead to positive social affiliations, whereas limited social acceptance may lead to aggression. Personalized instruction and cooperative learning enhances self-evaluation of intellectual competence.
3. Adolescence: Symbolic thought is used for self-regulation of antecedent behaviors, as more independence in daily activities requires planning ahead. Bodily changes, sexual urges, and intense relationships present a new challenge of self-management. Vicarious

learning can occur from appropriate modeling and incentives in impoverished environments.

4. Adulthood: People base their occupational choices for vocations upon their beliefs about self-knowledge, interests, and their ability to manage relationships. Technological trends in the workplace may require new skills. Environmental adaptations are enhanced through resiliency-based beliefs about one's self-efficacy. Transitions into parenting, spousal, and homemaking roles require efficacy adeptness to cultivate family values and manage careers. Midlife occupational balance of career efficacy may call for new habits and routines.

5. Maturity: Older adults reevaluate their physical efficacy for productivity and independence in daily activities. Targeted physical maintenance programs enhance cardiovascular efficacy, while increased emphasis on the utilization of cognitive and sociocultural activities offsets perceived physical inefficacy Bandura (1977b).

In regard to the development of self-efficacy across the life span, Bandura (1977b) emphasized that performance is the key to creating a person's belief, not only in their ability to accomplish an activity or participate in a relationship, but also in their coping ability to meet new challenges. Through their own behaviors, individuals develop adaptive skills and expectations that can be generalized to other situations, people, and places.

In his delineation about intervention for developmental change, Bandura (1977b) noted that "most treatment procedures developed in recent years to eliminate fearful and defensive behavior have been implemented either through performance or by symbolic procedures" (p. 198). Through a literature review, he characterized "attributional frameworks" (p. 199) that aim to reduce fear and anxiety about specific situations through symbolic visual images, as ineffectual; whereas in performance-based treatment strategies, people formulate expectancies about their capabilities, through experience. Bandura (1977b) used an "expectancy analysis" (p. 195) to delineate how activities will be planned so that they can be performed in graduated steps, as coherently tolerated and managed to result in self-efficacy.

Bandura suggested that the sense of resulting empowerment gained through successful performance is generalizable to other situations, which contain both a similar and a dissimilar type of threat (as the initial perceived fear). To test the construct validity of "efficacy expectations" (participant anticipation) to performance enactment of short-term goals, Bandura studied the effects of performance as a treatment for efficacy expectations. In a series of experiments designed to decease phobic fears, Bandura (1977b) demonstrated that people can significantly reduce their fears through performance modeling. People learn to believe in their performance, thereby changing their expectations of themselves for future anticipated activities. Although "vicarious" (observational) learning results were not as significant as the enactment of graduated activities aimed at fear reduction, both intervention methods were significantly more effective than the control group activities to enhance participation, thereby enhancing efficacy expectations (and decreasing phobic anxieties and activity avoidance) for future activities aimed at a specific context and goal.

The fit between Bandura's model and Llorens' theory. Although Bandura does not specifically state that the "adaptation process" is an inherent aspect of "doing" performance (Fidler & Fidler, 1978; King, 1978; Llorens, 1976), it is the cognitive recognition of productivity (both externally as a behavior and internally as a physiological-emotional arousal process) that provides an individual with self-efficacy beliefs. Indeed, it stands to reason that behavioral reorganization results from an adaptive occupational performance response (Llorens, 1991; Schultz & Schkade, 1992a, 1992b). Developmental mastery occurs as a result of an interaction of motivation with cognitive processes for improved occupational behavior self-regulation. Last, sociocultural beliefs in the determination of factors that facilitate healthy habits mobilize a person's inherent cognitive ability to willfully acquire new ways of thinking for developmental mastery and prevention of maladaptation (Bandura, 2004). People express these beliefs through the performance of occupational activities, tasks, and interpersonal relationships (Llorens, 1991). The author recommends the application of Bandura's developmental phases to Llorens' schematic in Part 3 of this issue.

Proposed Addition of Urie Bronfenbrenner's Concepts to Llorens' Theory

Next, the author analyzes Urie Bronfenbrenner's ecological theory of human development with corresponding life-span phases and compares his theory to Llorens' model for compatibility. Urie Bronfenbrenner's ecological systems theory (Brofenenbrenner, 1977, 1979, 2000; Bronfenbrenner & Morris, 1998) provides a bioecological developmental model (Bronfenbrenner & Ceci, 1994) of human development. Bronfenbrenner (1979) cited Lewin's gestalt field theory hypothesis: that behavior occurs as a function of a person's interaction with their environment: $B = f(PE)$ (p. 16). This concept elaborates upon the complex matrix of topographical interactions as biopsychosocial systems that enfold human development. This topological application of influences upon the growing person incorporates the concept of "motivational forces...emanating not from within the person but from the environment itself. Objects, activities, and especially other people send out lines of forces, valences, and vectors that attract and repel, thereby steering behavior and development" (Bronfenbrenner, 1979, p. 23). Bronfenbrenner (1979) represented the motivational forces that exist within various systems, as the (a) *microsystem*, which are the primary settings where individuals grow, develop, and interact, such as home, school, day care, clubs, shopping malls; (b) *mesosystem*, which are theoretical connectors or communicative links between the different primary settings (process wise); (c) *exosystem* are formal and informal environmental networks that influence, but do not contain, the growing person (community, government, parent work settings); and (d) *macrosystem*, which are the larger cultural prototype matrices that provide symbolic and ideological culture and sub-culture norms for growth and development. In a more recent publication, Bronfenbrenner added a fifth element to his model, called the (e) *chronosystem* (Bronfenbrenner, 2000), which delineates the passage of time; Llorens' theory already includes this aspect of temporality.

Bronfenbrenner used settings as a context to examine relationships, activities, and roles within and between settings. "The factors of place, time, physical features, activity, participant, and role constitute the elements of a setting" (Bronfenbrenner, 1977, p. 514). From this perspective, he stressed *process* as well as the content involved in the activity within and between settings to denote ecological relevancy to the growing person across the lifespan. In his identification of major settings and the ecological system relationships and their effects, Bronfenbrenner cited research of his own and others to explore and identify how ecological systems induce adaptation (Bronfenbrenner, 1977, 1979). Bronfenbrenner (1979) developed the concept of "ecological validity" (p. 28) to denote both naturalistic and experimental research, using the best of both worlds to capture the most representative "fit" between the individual and their environment.

In his description of the first property of an ecological setting, Bronfenbrenner used the term "reciprocity" (Bronfenbrenner, 1977, p. 519) to acknowledge the interplay of forces affecting both parties of a relationship. Second, he recognized the "functional social system" (p. 519). Viewing systems in this manner considers not only dyadic systems but also $N + 2$ systems that exert second- or higher-order effects. Therefore, triads and $N + 3$ systems can systematically influence behaviors of the people involved in both harmonious and negative ways, such as the effects of a positive spousal relationship on breastfeeding, or the effects of infant intervention in the NICU carrying over into the home, with increased reciprocity due to infant and caregiver enhancement in specific areas of growth and development. Additionally, sociocultural trends and activities affect the growing person, in addition to institutional values and mores that affect the meaning and motivation of particular activities, roles, and relationships.

Development and exercise of proximal processes in an ecology of human development. The author chose the following optimal "developmental outcomes" (italicized words only) directly from Bronfenbrenner and Ceci (1994, p. 569). These outcomes result from the interplay of an individual's biological endowments and the environment's facilitatory effects. Bronfenbrenner and Ceci (1994) described these developmental outcomes as *proximal processes* occurring in, or that influence contextual development in primary settings to reflect optimal ecological development in the actualization of a person's genetic potential (Bronfenbrenner & Ceci, 1994). The author constructed the age range and corresponding descriptions as approximations for each developmental phase based upon her knowledge of development and from an inferred progression in the literature (Bronfenbrenner & Ceci, 1994; also see Bronfenbrenner, 1977, 1979).

1. Infant: *Differentiated perception and response* (Bronfenbrenner & Ceci, 1994, p. 569). A child's perceptions about environmental organization (structure and function) affectively impact development through the perceptions of these elements upon the individual.

A child's developmental needs are addressed by significant others who interact with the child in daily activities. Dyads undergo change together because pairs have reciprocal relationships and mutually accommodate to each other. This accommodation results in the child's discrimination of his/her own actions needed for their role from those actions and properties of the sociocultural and physical environment.

2. Child: *Directing and controlling one's own behavior* (Bronfenbrenner & Ceci, 1994, p. 569). The child's behavior is initially directed from proximal environments that structurally interconnect one with the other. Functionally, children interact in a didactic manner in their interpersonal relationships and activities. This functional interaction favors a developmental reciprocity of meaningful activities guided by behavior role expectations.

3. Later childhood: *Coping successfully under stress* (Bronfenbrenner & Ceci, 1994, p. 569). Children learn to make "ecological transitions" (Bronfenbrenner, 1979, p. 6), or connections, between proximal environments as a function of the developmental process. The communication between ecological systems exerts an influence upon the participant's capacity to effectively symbolize, communicate about, and participate in novel contexts. This interaction of significant others in an interconnected capacity enhances generalizibility across primary and secondary environments, where the developing person assumes the balance of power to perform in these environments.

4. Adolescent: *Acquiring knowledge and skill* (Bronfenbrenner & Ceci, 1994, p. 569). The didactic nature of activities influences one's occupational (thoughtfulness needed for) role performance. A person's (occupational) role shapes their mental occupations (social cognition) about what they are thinking, and literally their physical, spatial, and temporal occupations regarding the form and performance in the occupation. Contextual activities occurring in specific roles are considered "molar" (1979, p. 46) or occupationally meaningful and volitional activities versus transient or accidental motor responses. Complex skills and behaviors develop as a function of these activities and relationships.

1. Young adult: *Establishing and maintaining mutually rewarding relationships* (Bronfenbrenner & Ceci, 1994, p. 569). A particular system of relationships exists within the function and structure

of a specific ecological environment. The dyad, or two-person system, establishes mutuality related to occupational activities and roles in the microsystem and exosystem. Maintenance of these dyadic relationships depends upon mesosystem interconnections between systems, including the macrosystem protocultural sphere, all of which include other structural entities (people, places, objects). These factors exert an influence upon the dyad; thus creating $N + 2$ systems.

2. Adult-maturity: *Modifying and constructing one's own physical, social, and symbolic environment* (Bronfenbrenner & Ceci, 1994, p. 569). The ability to mold the physical, social, and symbolic environment in a manner that is consistent with developmental needs, behaviors, and expectations for growth enables a mutual accommodation or adaptation to particular roles and purposeful activities. Adaptation to multiple settings, including cultural diversity, enhances "... cognitive competence and social skills" (1977, p. 212). The "power" connections one can establish to implement desired change (favorable to developing organisms) from primary to secondary settings and beyond enhance the developmental potential of these settings. The use of meaningful occupation and relationships within the occupational role determines the success of environmental modifications and construction.

The fit between Bronfenbrenner's model and Llorens' theory. Bronfenbronner (1977), like Llorens (1970, 1984a), believed that human beings have the capacity to "adapt and restructure their environments..." (Bronfenbrenner, 1977, p. 518). Bronfenbrenner also described human abilities as multidimensional and heuristic in nature, which means that research designs that do not consider the nested influence of ecological systems upon activities, relationships, and roles, will not effectively assess "... ecological structure and variation" (1977, p. 518). This interplay between mastery and environment correlates to the mutual reciprocity involved in Section 3 of Llorens (1970) theory of "Behavior Expectations and Adaptive Skills" (p. 97), which "... from a developmental perspective, [must] identify the processes of mutual accommodation between a growing organism and its changing surround" (Bronfenbrenner, 1977, p. 518). The environments in which humans occupy themselves must contain activities, and those environments that are indirectly associated with these environments must be considered as interconnected systems to determine the behavior expectations and adaptive skills necessary for developmental mastery (Bronfenbrenner & Morris, 1998). The author applies Bronfenbrenner's developmental phases for ecological growth and development in Part 3 of this issue.

Proposed Addition of Jerome Brunner to Llorens' Theory

The last new theorist for consideration is Jerome Brunner, whose extensive work into the growth of intellect and the role of adaptation to one's habitat crosses the boundaries of both Bandura's self-efficacy and Bronenbrenner's ecology of human development. Jerome Bruner's "discovery learning" paradigm (Driscoll, 1994, p. 218) draws from a developmental constructivist framework that is based upon Piaget's schemas of intellectual growth (Bruner, 1965, 1966, 1975, 1976). Discovery learning is described as both a psychological "theory of [cognitive] growth" (Bruner, 1966, p. 5) and as a type of learning instruction (Bruner, 1966; Driscoll, 1994). Bruner constructed three developmental stages that encompass growth processes or modes of thinking. A child passes through these stages in their maturation of understanding abstract thought. Whereas Piaget described the epistemological aspects of cognitive growth (Bruner, 1966), Bruner added the psychological processes related to a child's developmental progression, beginning with the motor learning ability required to interactively manipulate models to the mental capacity to represent designs and visual images, and finally to the use of language and mathematical symbols (Bruner, 1965, 1966, 1975, 1976).

Bruner explained cognitive growth activities as a process model in the "growth sciences" (Bruner, 1965, p. 1016). In addition to drawing from the neurobehavioral and social sciences, he used the concept of activity theory to formulate these growth stages because activities encompass the duality of thought and action in multiple spheres of science (Bruner, 1966), as activity subroutines through play (Bruner, 1973). He proposed six mediating processes to support his hypothesized theory of cognitive growth that occur during everyday activities and interactions.The author paraphrases these six mediating processes as (a) habituation to stimuli and selection of attention for repetition and variation, (b) memory schemas to store these experiences, (c) communication of personal orientation and intended navigation, (d) learning through appropriate guidance, (e) language as a tool to organize time and space, and that (f) purposeful activities demand multiple simultaneous aspects of mental occupation (Bruner, 1966, pp. 5–6).

Bruner posited that cognitive processes developed during the evolutionary course of hominids when a more upright posture allowed for the development of manipulative skills. As children mature, modes of categorical thinking and causal relationships evolve through the use of hand functions in relationship with affective objective relationships. Bruner depicted the importance of play as practice in mastery; through play, children subjectively explore how their culture communicates about mores, values, and morals (Bruner, 1965, 1976). Communication occurs through the activities that children observe. "Children, besides, are constantly playing imitatively with the rituals, implements, tools, and weapons of the adult world" (Bruner, 1965, p. 1008). Through spontaneous exploration and experimentation, cognitive processes mature, allowing children to learn how and why adults use various tools in their engagement of a daily round of occupational activities. Brunner suggested that the types of motor and language skills used in a child's daily activities developed as tools of thought that reflect these cognitive processes (Bruner, 1966, 1975). Activities involve action sequences with the hands that permit thoughtful exploration and learning discovery. Bruner suggested that his theory of cognitive development be utilized as a problem-based approach to educational instruction (Bruner, 1966).

The author bases the following stages of cognitive-constructive development upon Bruner (1965, 1966, 1973).

1. Infor: *Enactive stage* (approximately 0–3 years): This stage of cognitive growth encompasses the function (*F*) of (ab) above in the mediating process model. Development of intelligence during this stage incorporates the use of agent-object "segments of action [which] are, in effect, positions *occupied* [italics added] in a sequence..." (Brunner, 1975, p. 13), including interpersonal relationships. Children manipulate, resolve, and guide actions through purposeful activity, as schematic sequences, from beginning to end. Examples include construction of simple models and building, moving through mazes, games, drawing, all daily activities, including feeding one's self, bathing, dressing, combing hair, brushing teeth, and imaginative play such as peek-a-boo, hide

and seek, talking on the telephone (as an action or as a pretend action).

2. Child: *Iconic stage* (approximately 3–8 years): This stage of cognitive growth incorporates the use of representational images and designs as a *F*(cd) above. "Images develop an autonomous status, they become great summarizers of action" (Brunner, 1966, p. 13). Visual memory for concrete objects and relationships occurs in the form of representational drawings of objects (houses, people, things, animals, places), maps, arrangement of food items on plate, blocks, or pick-up sticks. Bruner noted "...the image of the moment is sufficient and it is controlled by a single feature of the situation" (Brunner, p. 13). Occupational mediation of schematic formation relegates like images to like schema structures.

3. Later childhood: *Symbolic stage* (beginning approximately 8 years—developing through adulthood): This stage of cognitive growth incorporates the use of symbols to express abstract concepts and involves the *F*(dc) above. The use of logic and reasoning in relationship to the self permits the use of language as a tool "...for translating experience [through occupational associations] into more powerful systems for notation and ordering" (Brunner, 1966, p. 21). Examples of process-oriented occupational activities include the employment of "thought processes, ways of thinking that employ language and formation of explanation, and later use of such languages as mathematics and logic and even automatic servants to crank out the consequences" (Bruner, 1965, p. 1009). These activities are also grouped schematically as occupational tasks used in productive or leisure role activities such as work, self-care, learning tasks, play and leisure, as relegated by culture.

As an instructional method. Bruner explained the potential of discovery based learning in the following manner.

> We shall, of course, try to encourage students to discover on their own. Children need not discover all generalizations for themselves, obviously. Yet we want to give them the opportunity...to operate independently. ...For if we do nothing else, we should somehow give to children a respect for their own powers of thinking..." (Bruner, 1966, p. 96).

Brunner cited Vygotsy's theory of activity-based learning (Bruner, 1966) and developed the idea of "scaffolding" (Bruner, 1975, p. 12) to reflect the support that can be given to assist children to make the connection between the enactive, representational, and symbolic levels of cognition. These methods of problem-solving may occur in one activity for people of all ages throughout the lifespan, as each phase provides intention and feedback, "and the patterns of action that mediate between them [within and between phases]" (Bruner, 1973, p. 1). The use of scaffolding in discovery learning is analogous to Vygotsky's concept of *proximal zones of development* (Bruner, 1975), in that the mode of presentation of materials can serve as a beginning level of instruction needed for later, more complex and abstract thinking skills. Bruner posited that learners need for self-reflection and internalized understanding of how a subject relates to the learner is important. Because, to ". . . personalize knowledge . . . one makes the familiar an instance of a more general case and thereby produces awareness of it" (p. 1015), resulting in "self-conscious reflectiveness" (p. 1015). By moving through a process of discovery learning, children learn . . . "that it is alright to entertain and express highly subjective ideas to treat a task as a problem where you *invent* an answer rather than *finding* one out there in the book or on the blackboard" (p. 1014).

Bruner (1999) concluded his synopsis about growth and development with a narrative about infancy, culture, and the intersubjectivity that encumbers all learning, as infants watch the intention of others. Culture requires this sensitivity where intention and meaning blend into intentionality as a discriminatory (activity) analysis about how to interpret objects and symbols. Mutual expectancies are developed through the process of enculturation.

The fit between Bruner's discovery learning model with Llorens' theory. Bruner described the enormous potential of schools to provide students a kind of instruction to free them from the nuances of completing every experience of everyday life to find meaning in learning, and of mundane memorization of meaningless facts, by amplifying appropriate skills to scaffold progressively complex cognitive skills. Discovery learning methods involve the progression of interactive experience, from manipulation of models to designs of visual images, to language and mathematical symbols. In much the same fashion as Llorens, Bruner used the concept of mastery in the development of behavior expectation and adaptive skills to provide learners with the problem-solving tools they need for an optimum growth experience. The author recommends Jerome Bruner's *Discovery Learning* paradigm for inclusion into Llorens' theory and applies his developmental phases in Part 3 of this issue.

Discussion of Bandura, Bronfenbrenner, and Bruner as Related to Llorens' Theory

Bruner (1976) remarked that ". . . one cannot easily separate the cognitive from the connotative and the affective" (Bruner, 1976, p. 31). In her model of *Facilitating Growth and Development . . .*, Llorens (1970) accomplished this feat. By linking together the concept of activity components in Section 1, as "mastery of particular skills, abilities, and relationships in each of the areas of neurophysiological, physical, psychosocial, and psychodynamic development, social language, daily living, and sociocultural skills . . . to the successful achievement of satisfactory coping behavior and adaptive relationships . . ." (Llorens, 1970, p. 94), and the influences of the environment in Section 3, as ". . . the stimulation of experiences received within the environment of the family . . . [and] later the influences of extended family, community, social and civic groups [which] assist in the growth process (p. 94)," Llorens' theoretical delineations of growth and development achieved the correlation of the cognitive, with the connotative and the affective (Bruner, 1976). In addition to these two explanatory sections about how humans develop mastery as means (Section 1) and ends (Section 3) during the growth process, she also predicted, in Section 2, how and why the occupational therapist uses activities (occupation) and personal relationships. This section stands upon the basis that occupational performance, enabled through Section 1 activity components of sensorimotor integration, and appropriate affective object relationships, will lead to Section 3 occupational role behavior in meaningful contexts. She illustrated this continuum in facilitating selected activities and relationships of Section 2 as a linkage between enablement of performance (as a process) to occupational synchronicity (as person-occupation-environment balance). Bronfenbrenner's concept of mesosystem linkage as a connector to all other bioecological systems correlates to Llorens' systems thinking of process and product, joined by specific kinds of occupational activities and relationships.

Last, Llorens' emphasis upon occupational performance, which incorporates *doing as engagement*, is certainly consistent with Bandura's performance-based theory of social learning and health promotion.

Rosenburg (2000) described the value of a theory according to it's simplicity and economy. These tenets are reflected in the three inter-related sections of Llorens' theory as *Developmental Expectations, Behaviors and Needs; Facilitating Activities and Relationships;* and *Behavior Expectations and Adaptive Skills.* As noted by Llorens, this complex model was never meant to serve as a recipe or cookbook application. Indeed, health care practitioners must be familiar with each of the growth models presented; rather, Llorens' model serves as a guide to illustrate what Royeen (2003) noted as "occupational shaping" (p. 617)—the developmentally based process that shapes humans in context with their environments. Through this shaping, many factors act simultaneously at specific times, and temporally, as human's age, to culminate in a human being.

Conclusion of Part 1

Part 1 of this review, update, and theoretical expansion of Llorens introduced the reader to *The Developmental Theory of Occupational Therapy*, including the thesis, the theoretical premises, and the model for practice. After an analysis of the changes and updates Llorens made to her model, the author evaluated the need for further change. Through an extensive literature review, it was determined that the psychodynamics section needed revision to reflect Freud's emphasis upon the paradigm of centrally generated patterns in erogenous zone maturation, with the development of affective object relationships as corollary occupational activities and relationships. A motivational theory of character development (Peck & Havighurst, 1960) was analyzed and synthesized as a companion to the psychosexual development component. Finally, the author analyzed and synthesized growth models of three additional theorists, Albert Bandura, Urie Bronfenbrenner, and Jerome Brunner, for application into the Llorens model to further update and expand upon her basic concepts of mastery and adaptation in occupational performance components, activities and relationships, and roles during the growth process. The application of these concepts and theorists in Part 3 provides an enhanced schematic and revised premises of *Facilitating Growth and Development...*, based upon

Llorens (1991), to build a practice and process model for occupational therapy services in the NICU. This concludes Part 1 of this issue.

PART 2: OCCUPATIONAL PHYSIOLOGY

In the second component, or Part 2, of this book, the author addresses current research in human development regarding the concept of endogenously generated motor activity for age specific occupational performance. In particular, this section analyzes and synthesizes current research about genetically encoded central pattern sequences of movement to satisfy specific affective and object developmental demands (Llorens, 1991). This synthesis provides support for the inherent value of purposeful activities (occupation) and relationships in the spatiotemporal and occupational adaptation processes as a product of *occupational physiology*. Last, as an example of application, the author discusses infant vulnerability as related to neuroplasticity and synchronicity for infant and family adaptation in the NICU.

Adaptive Occupation Begins with Purposeful Activity Sequences

The Central Pattern Generator Concept

Heinz Prechtl, scientist and neonatalogist, conjectured that infants endogenously generate motor activity for age-specific (occupational) performance (Prechtl, 1997). He noted that movement sequences or patterns are genetically encoded and endogenously expressed for the purpose of specific developmental demands or *ontogenetic adaptation* (Prechtl, 2001). One consequence of ontogenetic adaptation is that, at different phases of the lifespan, as proposed in prominent theories of human development, the function and structure of the central nervous system is morphologically different.

Research regarding the concept of central pattern generators provides depth to theories of human growth and development. Erik von Holst (1973) and others have proposed underlying neurophysiological mechanisms that support humankind's drive for mastery and competence throughout the lifespan. Prechtl (1997) supports his views on development and, in particular, ontogenetic adaptation through his exploration of the central pattern generator phenomena.

Prechlt (1997) cited von Holst (1973) to explain neuroplasticity and ontogenetic adaptation through the central pattern generator paradigm and its relationship to the physiology of activity.

Erich van Holst spent his experimental life's work on what he called 'Zentrale Automatie' (central automatism) (1973) and what is now called 'central pattern generator' (CPG). It is only during the last decade that we have reached a better understanding of the cellular and molecular mechanism responsible for endogenously generated motor activity . . . (Prechtl, 1997, p. 5).

Life cycles, both human and animal, include circadian rhythms, elements of innate motor control, and rhythmic neuroendocrine functions which regulate reproductive status (Kandel, Schwartz, & Jessell, 1995). According to Llorens (1970, 1976, 1991), a combination of developmental processes or activity components blend together to satisfy an individual's developmental expectations, behaviors, and needs to meet contextual occupational demands in a dynamic person-occupation-environment transaction (Llorens, 1986). The mechanisms that "drive" these transactions for ontogenetic adaptation to explain the occupational physiology of sensorimotor integration have come to be known as central pattern generators (Arshavsky, 2003; Arshavsky, Deliagina, & Orlovsky, 1997; Benjamin, Staras, & Kemenes, 2000; Bjorklund, 1997; Cohen, 1999; Commissiong, Sauve, Csonka, Karoum, & Toffano, 1991; Fenelon, Casasnovas, Simmers, & Meyrand, 1998; Graybiel, 1997; Grillner, Markram, DeSchutter, Silberberg, & Le Beau, 2005; Kemenes, Staras, &Benjamin, 2001; Kiehn & Kullander, 2004; Kuo, 2002; Lydic, 1989; Marder & Bucher, 2001; Silberberg, & LeBeau, 2005; Staras, Kemenes, Benjamin, & Kemenes, 2003; von Holst, 1973; Yuste, MacLean, Smith, & Lansner, 2005).

Central Pattern Generation Across The Lifespan

Functional Significance of Central Pattern Generators

Central pattern generators (CPGs) consist of both individual neuronal cell groupings, or cell assemblies, and neuronal networks (Arshavsky, 2003; Grillner et al., 2005; Yuste et al., 2005). They are found at all levels of the brain and spinal cord (Marder & Bucher,

2001) and are physiologically capable of producing rhythmical neuronal patterns that culminate in purposeful activities (Cotterill, 2000, 2001; Dubbeldam, 2001; Graybiel, 1997; von Holst, 1973). Although CPGs can generate rhythmical activity in the absence of sensory input (von Holst, 1973), the CPG is present across species for species-specific adaptation, both phylogenetically and ontogenetically, and depend upon internal and external sensory stimuli for entrainment of the CPG (Cohen, 1992). The role of sensory stimuli

FIGURE 5. The Role of Sensory Stimuli in CPG Function. Illustration from Cohen (1992). The Bottom Figure Illustrates the Old View About How CPGs Operated to Provide Efferent Muscle and Limb Movement, with Hierarchical Influence from Command Centers and a Sensory Relay Feedback Loop. The Top Figure Illustrates Newer Views of the Emergent and Distributed Properties of the Heterarchial Control Involved in Purposive Action (reproduced with permission)

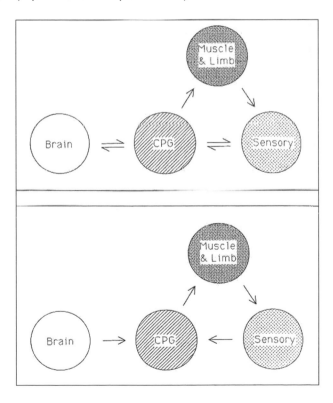

in the formation of CPG functioning has vastly changed the conceptual model about how CPG assemblies and networks integrate input for adaptation. Figure 5 illustrates the changes in thinking regarding the role of sensory stimuli in the emergent and distributed function attributed to CPGs.

Interestingly, CPGs filter their incoming sensory input to decrease distortion and thereby improve accuracy (Kemenes et al., 2001; Kuo, 2002). Neurophysiologists initially studied cellular preparations of rhythmical pattern generation in invertebrates, such as giant axons in squid, and ganglia in snails and lobsters. These cellular networks were relatively easy to isolate, observe, and stimulate for causal analysis. For example, in the pond snail *Lymnaea* a well-identified rhythmic CPG drives motor neurons for feeding-related musculature activity sequences (Benjamin et al., 2000). Interestingly, the motivational state of the animal, in regard to hunger or satiation, influences the expression of feeding and respiratory behaviors via sensory integratory input to modulatory interneurons of the CPG. Both operant and classical conditioning influences the feeding and respiratory responses. Learning and memory changes demonstrated plasticity by the strength of synaptic and neurotransmitter connectivity and content in regard to (a) presynaptic sub-threshold response to the sensory input, and (b) the long-term facilitation of the synaptic input's amplitude as measured in the excitatory post-synaptic potential. These responses were illustrated through electrophysiological parameters of prepared specimens. Interestingly, Staras et al. (2003) demonstrated in the same creature that a singular CPG network, which regulates feeding, is controlled by tonic and phasic inhibition of the CPG's rhythmic behavior. In the absence of food, the feeding movements involved in lip and rasping movements are tonically inhibited. However, when food is present, the neurons that provide the tonic inhibitory input to the whole CPG are switched to a phasic firing mode. This switch provides the necessary phasic inhibitory inputs that, in conjunction with electrophysiological plateaus of depolarization in another CPG neuron type, make the system capable of varied responses to environmental stimuli such as is present in the smell and taste of food. Kemenes et al. (2006) found that persistent depolarization of the soma of a modulatory neuron provides a nonsynaptic formation of long-term memory, and may provide a back-up system to CPG synaptic circuits. These neurons are extrinsic to the intrinsic feeding neural circuitry and recruit and encode associative learning in the intrinsic neurons for long-term memory of the snail's feeding behavioral network.

Studies in cats, rabbits, dogs, and monkeys verified the existence of centrally patterned rhythmical generation in mammals (Cohen, 1999; von Holst, 1973). Kiehn and Kullander (2004) noted the use of genetics to decipher how genes influence the cellular and membrane characteristics of CPGs. In "a dialogue between genes and synapses," Kandel (2006, p. 261) explained that new synaptic connections are entrained by environmental stimuli through sensitization, association, or habituation, thus leading to long-term memory consolidation. Long-term memory occurs through specific synapses that are marked for synaptic growth when molecular and genetic encoding facilitates long-term potentiation or depression through experience or practice. Long-term potentiation/depression in mammals is compared to long-term facilitation/inhibition, respectively, for invertebrates.

CPG Development

During gestational development, CPG cellular groupings appear in the spinal cord and brain stem by seven weeks gestational age (Fenelon et al., 1998), producing spontaneous fetal movements. However, little is known about the development of CPGs from infancy through adulthood. According to Fenelon et al. (1998), the final architecture of CPGs varies considerably from that seen in infancy, indicating that specific changes take place in CPG architecture during the developmental process. Developmental phases in the development of CPGs support earlier behaviors other than the final end-stage behavior, and therefore play a crucial role in the developmental process, as illustrated in Llorens' (1991) schematic. In addition, specific behaviors that will eventually be expressed by specific CPGs during development are silent during certain developmental phases, even though the CPG is structurally intact and capable of functioning. This indicates that CPGs play an important role in critical periods in the development of species-specific behaviors.

During critical periods of specific developmental phases, the establishment of CPG synaptic connections and structural properties of nerve cells undergo dynamic changes for enhanced connectivity that are typical of maturation for that age period (Bjorklund, 1997; Fenelon et al., 1998). The central pattern generation in the fetus and newborn are the result of intra-CPG connectivity and membrane properties in relationship to other functional CPG assemblies and networks, "...not withstanding late developmental tuning and synaptic wiring..." (Fenelon et al., 1998, p. 707). The ability for CPG cellular networks to generate rhythmicity develops from this synaptic connectivity and through the redistribution of genetic cellular material incorporated into the cellular membrane (Arshavsky, 2003; Marder & Bucher, 2001).

The coordination of various CPGs for occupational task purposes within the contingency of specific ecological contexts occurs through an occupational selection process allowing emergent and distributive dynamic systems within the CNS to adapt to change (Arshavsky, 2003; Graybiel, 1997; Pearson, 2000; Redgrave, Prescott, & Gurney, 1999). Sensorimotor action sequences underlie cognitive occupational physiologic processes, such as declarative memory storage, language functions, and visual spatial skills, as well as interpersonal skills, perceptual discrimination, and ego adaptive functions (Bruner, 1973; Cotterill, 2000, 2001; Kandel et al., 1995; Llorens, 1970; Llorens & Rubin, 1962, 1967). Last, pattern generation between functional CPG systems are hypothesized to exist as loops within the CNS (Graybiel, 1997; Lewis, 1997; Redgrave et al., 1999).

The concept of receptive fields, whereby a neuron is excited by a specific type of sensory input, encouraged a Hebbian view of sensory systems; stimuli that are survival serving are rewarding (reinforced). These stimuli are wired together genetically and are inherently attractive (attractors) for occupational engagement. The CPG concept could explain the specific kinds of neuromodulators, protein synthesis, and endocrine chemical relationships necessary to transcribe sensory data to successfully input object-action-sequences (Johansson, 1998). These CPG systems include cooperation between such structures as the supplementary and premotor cortices, limbic system (amygdala and hippocampus), basal ganglia, cerebellum, hypothalamus, brain stem (Cotterill, 2000, 2001; Grillner, 2005), and spinal cord (lumbo- and cervicothoracal areas) (Dubbeldam, 2001; Zehr et al., 2004). Sensory input shapes the patterned activity output during the course of daily occupations and provides a signaling function during specific critical periods across the life span (Arshavsky, 2003; Fenelon et al., 1998; Kandel et al., 1995). Developmentally, sensory input entrains the CPG to anticipate movement patterns in the entire system. Although these CPG systems are evolutionarily (morphologically) different, "...these circuits also function as substrates for the integration of sensory input" (Yuste et al., 2005, p. 478). Rhythmical pattern generation is robust in the early stages of development and continues throughout life (Marder & Bucher, 2001).

Emergent and Distributed Systems: CPG Mechanisms and the Dynamics of Neurochaos

Neurological Landmarks

Figures 6 and 7 illustrate many (but not all) of the neurological structures referred to in the CPG literature. The concept of heterarchial CPG systems provides support for the concept of activity theory, where an individual's moment-to-moment occupational demands afford the maximal degrees of freedom for a rich repertoire of activity choices (Bernstein, 1967; Brooks, 1986). Phylogenetically and ontogenetically, the topography and structural aspect of CPG systems drives the functional aspect of pattern generation within a specific neurological area, and may also represent localized functions such as seen in face recognition, declarative memory, speech production, and language comprehension (Arshavsky, 2003), in addition to the more global and distributed functions previously discussed. And the changes initiated in the CPG assemblies, in either the more focal or globally distributed functions, are very likely propagated by non-linear dynamical and neurochaotic mechanisms (Cohen, 1992; Korn & Faure, 2003) (see Figure 6).

Lewis, Caldwell, and Barker (2003) cited the following abbreviations for Figure 7: "CN, caudate nucleus; GPe, globus pallidus, external segment; GPi, globus pallidus, internal segment; SNc, substantia nigra pars compacta; SNr, substantia nigra pars reticulata; (p. 2)." For the sake of clarification, the authors did not illustrate the GPe/SNr connection with the Caudate Nucleus. The various arrows indicate the fiber tract connections. Their corresponding neuro-transmitters are not shown here.

CPG Mechanics

The variety of behaviors that humans exhibit is possible due to a coupling of intra- and inter-CPG properties, producing a coordinated

Lynne F. La Corte

FIGURE 6. Mapping the Brain. Illustration by Lewis Calver, Biomedical Communications, The University of Texas Southwestern Medical Center at Dallas (reproduced with permission)

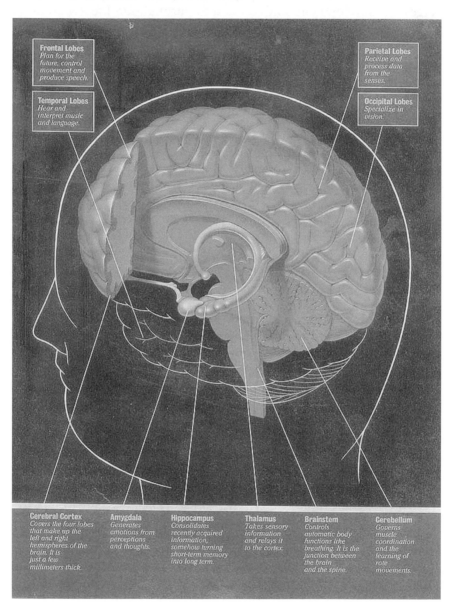

FIGURE 7. The Basal Ganglia. From Lewis, Caldwell, and Barker (2003) (reproduced with permission)

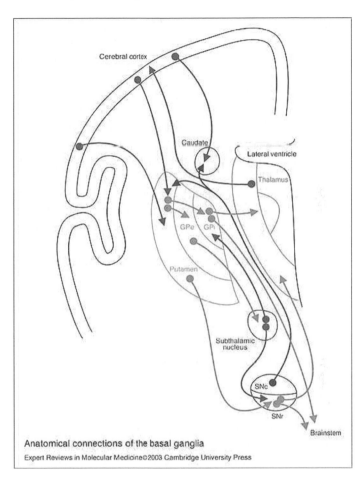

Anatomical connections of the basal ganglia
Expert Reviews in Molecular Medicine©2003 Cambridge University Press

effort of synchronized CPG cell assemblies in a unified manner to produce complex behaviors. The rhythmic aspect of behavioral patterns, resulting from coordination among the various CPGs, allows body segments to be used individually for a greater degree of species adaptation (Bem, Cabelguen, Ekeberg, & Grillner, 2003; Dubbeldam, 2001; Marder & Bucher, 2001). Marder and Bucher (2001) noted that the underlying mechanism for pattern generation depend upon the "...strength, time course, and time-dependent properties" (p. 988) of the synaptic connections, the intrinsic cellular membrane properties, and the phasing and frequency of pattern generation within the CPG cellular networks.

Additionally, Marder and Bucher (2001) relayed that the cycle period, the burst duration which initiates a cycle, the duty cycle (burst duration/cycle period), and phase of firing of an individual unit of pattern generation (delay between cycles/cycle period) can be used to quantify central pattern generation of a specific kind of rhythmic pattern. The two main mechanisms for rhythm production are the pacemaker neurons and the cell assemblies whose synaptic properties generate rhythms. Pacemaker or core oscillator neurons excite other neurons to fire in a rhythm, and these neurons are found in the vertebrate respiratory cycle as an arousal mechanism (Marder & Bucher, 2001), and also in the basal ganglia (program selector of occupation) (Redgrave et al., 1999), hypothalamus (neuroendocrine and circadian rhythms), and hippocampus (memory retention) (Kandel, 2006; Kandel et al., 1995).

The other mechanism used in cellular assemblies for pattern generation is reciprocal inhibition, which is also known as a "half center oscillator" (Marder & Bucher, 2001, p. 989). This mechanism works through coupling, where one neuron inhibits another as membrane properties of spike frequency adapt with the consequent release of inhibitory neurotransmitter. This kind of pattern generation can be found in the cerebellum (Kandel et al., 1995). In particular, the cerebellum oscillatory system exhibits five times the latency of the cortex and is completely inhibitory. Therefore, the cerebellum is highly involved in long-term potentiation and depression in an oscillatory feed-forward manner, which provides a spatiotemporal timing mechanism for learning and memory (Grillner et al., 2005). Importantly, the *transitions* between half center oscillators, in regard to periodicity, occur through alternation of inhibition and excitation (Marder & Bucher, 2001). Marder and Bucher also noted that, as the inhibitory effects of one cell body upon another decline, the reciprocal neuron's membrane potential becomes excitatory, consequently inhibiting its coupled partner. This coupling of inhibitory reciprocity generates a rhythmical pattern, "... providing a core feature in almost all known central patterning generation networks..." (p. 989). As previously mentioned, "loss of self-inhibition is a cellular mechanism for episodic rhythmic behavior" (Staras et al., 2003, p. 116).

Structurally, central pattern generators connect with or consist of premotor neurons that drive motor neurons, or the motor neurons may be part of or directly connected to the CPG. Additionally, neuromodulation of CPGs occurs through the release of neuromodulator substances, hormones, and sensory transmitters to act upon the release of neurotransmitter, such as glutamate. These substances work in parallel to facilitate, inhibit, stimulate, or motivate (prime) CPGs. The modulation of CPGs may occur through descending pathways, ascending afferent fibers from the periphery or from glandular secretions of hormones. Neuromodulators affect "the synaptic strength and intrinsic membrane properties" (Marder & Bucher, 2001, p. 990) in the frequency and phasing of the CPG units. In addition, there is evidence that several different pattern generators may work together to affect the coordination of various activity components that are involved in occupation.

Understanding neuromodulation is important because phasically timed sensory input activates neuromodulator substances (Arshavsky, 2003). In cases of neurotrauma, such as spinal cord injury, the effects of embryonic raphe neurons on lumbar CPG activity in the spinal cord may be enhanced by the neurotransmittor serotonin through new routes, which in turn modulate the generation of rhythmical movement (Commissiong et al., 1991; y Ribotta et al., 2000; also see Jacobs & Fornal, 1997).

Neurochaos within CPG Systems

According to Korn and Faure (2003), chaos theory explains how the human organism uses central pattern generation to accomplish important goals from an evolutionary perspective to include tasks requiring the cognitive processes, information processing and memory, pattern recognition, and recall. The brain uses purposeful and meaningful movement to creatively integrate relevant perceptual data into memory as a self-organizing process (Korn & Faure, 2003).

In fact, in an intervertabrate (lobster) stomatogastric ganglion, synaptic plasticity is dependent upon the sensory dynamics of CPG neurons (Korn & Faure, 2003). Discharges are demonstrated in shifts of *in* and *out of phase* oscillations, typical of external sensory systems, and ". . . were maintained in the reset state until a new signal was received" (p. 805). In regard to the role of dynamical chaotic systems,

Korn and Faure (2003) noted that "... a single network can subserve several different functions and participate in more than one behavior ... the functional organization of the network can be substantially modified ... and are still able to generate oscillatory antiphasic [chaotic] patterns" (p. 801). From a behavioral and biological standpoint, the *in* and *out of phase* of synchronized oscillations (through inhibitory and excitatory modulatory effects) serves to allow for adaptation through a quick adjustment to synchronicity from unstable chaotic systems. Changing environments require quick transitional movements and behaviors that can be resynchronized through different couplings of chaotic cellular assemblies. In this manner, activity components needed for biological and behavioral goals, in accordance with occupational demands and intrinsic motivation, can be associated. The chaos model proposes a readiness system based upon specific task attributes. Intrinsic motivation enables the selection and activation of activity components to emerge as novel or anticipated occupational associations for occupational engagement of familiar or new activity patterns.

Since neurochaos has been reported throughout the brain and spinal cord, and CPG elements act as distributed and emergent programs, self-organized (chaotic) activity patterns, based upon perceptual schema are generated by the brain for environmental adaptation (Korn & Faure, 2003). This thought was also stated by von Holst (1973), who noted that "The human mind always wants to order its environment" (p. 220). According to von Holst's theory of automatisms, the *in* and *out of phase* rhythmical pattern oscillators "represent the form in which one automatism fights for control of the other" (p. 26), reflecting what von Holst called the *magnet effect*, which "is the endeavor of one automatism to impose its tempo and a quite specific reciprocal phase relationship upon another" (p. 25). "Coordination [of automatisms] is not fixed and machine like, but variable, flowing and plastic" (p. 31). Furthermore, two or three automatisms can be superimposed upon each other to "provide[s] 'associations' in the truest sense of the word between different central processes, which are in principal independent" (p. 63–64). Thus, an additive effect of occupation activity components follows chaotic theory (magnet effect) for "absolute coordination" (p. 27) of distributed and emergent systems. Interestingly, von Holst noted that he used the words "magnet effect" descriptively to represent a "mechanical coupling through a viscous medium [and would do so]... until the physical process in the CNS... is more clearly understood" (p. 73). According to von Holst (1973), when activity components are added together, as automatisms, a specific frequency relationship of the superimposed component rhythms can be visualized. He noted "... even under normal conditions quite arrhythmic, specific 'reflexes' are similarly based upon automatic-rhythmic processes, such as the respiratory and locomotor rhythms, but that their activity is modified to a tremendous extent by stimuli and central impulses. (Consider, for example, the enormous distortion of the rhythmic medullary respiratory impulses imposed by human speaking and singing)" (p. 116). von Holst (1973), Korn and Faure (2003), and others have observed the processes involved in the coordination of neural networks. von Holst described the magnetic effect that pulls together, as recruitment, the coordination of relevant synaptic pathways needed to meet specific internal and external conditions; whereas Korn and Faure described this process as chaotic, whereby this coordination can be variable and therefore versatile.

For order to emerge from chaos, the author speculates in support of Llorens' hypothesis of the inherent value of activity (occupational theory). Purposeful and meaningful occupational forms, relationships, and environments must be recognized via their sensory properties as intrinsically and extrinsically motivating and reinforcing, or in the alternative, as avoidance. In this manner, the anticipation of meaningful activity unites the revelant CPG networks to exert a novel and organizing effect upon the brain.

Occupational Physiology

Functional CPG Systems

Although neurochaos provides a mechanism for central pattern generation, it does not provide a framework for structural coordination within and between CPG systems. Josephine Moore, occupational therapy neuroanatomy professor extraordinaire, provided such a framework to explain how activity components, through evolution, became coupled as distributed and emergent systems. Moore adapted Paul T. MacLean's (1973) triune brain theory (Gilfoyle et al., 1990). This theory divides the brain into three phylogenetic periods: the (a) archi system (oldest), (b) paleo system (moderately old), and (c) the neo and neo-neo system (newer). This theory can also be viewed as functional CPG archi, paleo, and neo systems in regard to a person's occupations, because each system contains CPGs involving (a) archi homeostatic behaviors (visceral, endocrine functions, and circadian rhythms), attention in wakefulness, rest, or sleep, and orientation to time and space; (b) paleo emotional regulation and balance, patterns of locomotion, orientation to visual, auditory, and somatosensory stimuli, protection, and the development of affective responses; and (c) neo and neo-neo exploratory/discrimina-criminatory skills, reflective, skillful, intellectual, creative and artistic endeavors (Gilfoyle et al., 1990).

According to Moore (Gilfoyle et al., 1990), there are seven functional structural areas, each of which contains a combination of the archi, paleo, and neo system dimensions or activity components for occupational performance (Llorens, 1976) and spatiotemporal adaptation (Gilfoyle et al., 1990). Figure 8 depicts the archi, paleo, and neo system relationships for each structural area.

These structural areas, depicted by Moore (Gilfoyle et al., p. 41) are as follows.

1. Spinal cord
2. Brain stem—medulla
3. Brain stem—pons
4. Brain stem—midbrain
5. Cerebellum
6. Thalamus
7. Cerebral hemispheres

Archi, Paleo, and Neo Systems in Central Pattern Generation

Growth and development in the seven major structural areas is based upon Moore (Gilfoyle et al., 1990). The phlogenetically older archi structures develop first, followed by, and overlapping with the intermediate level paleo structures. The newer brain structures develop last; this includes the neo-cortex system and the neo-neo frontal lobe with its connections to important subcortical structures. Moore noted that there is a tremendous amount of overlap in the development of these areas, with intermediate and newer systems exerting increasingly more modulation as myelination and central pattern generation proceeds in an ontogenetically adaptive manner.

FIGURE 8. Moore's Seven Functional Structural Areas of the Brain. A Characteristic Diagram of Moore's CNS Art Work from Gilfoyle et al. (1990). This Illustration Portrays the Concept of the Three Systems within the Seven Structural Areas of the CNS as the (a) Older (Archi), (b) Intermediate (Paleo), and (c) Neo (Newer) Areas of the Brain and Spinal Cord, Each of which is Included in All of the Seven Major Structural Units within the Central Nervous System (Reproduced with Permission). (See Table 4 for mnemonics)

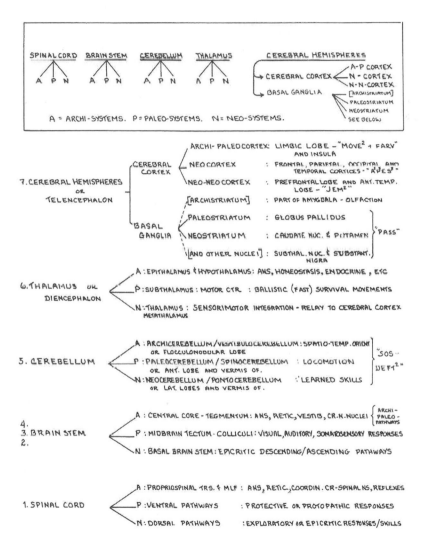

TABLE 4. Key to Moore's Mnemonics

Key	These Mnemonics are Based Upon Moore; from Gilfoyle et al. (1990), p. 61
MOVE^2 (*sic*) M^{2}OVE	Motivation and memory circuits, Olfaction, visceral, emotional tone (limbic system)
FARV	Fear, anger, rage, violence (limbic system)
A^{2}P^{2}ES^3	Appreciates and anticipates, plans, programs and executes skills and survival stratagems (neocortical system)
JEM^2	Judgment, emotional tone, motivation, memory circuits (neo-neo cortical system)
PASS	Postural and/or movement, adaptations as stereotyped or semi-automatic learned responses (basal ganglion as background movement patterns)
SOS-DEFT^2	Smooth and orderly sequencing of (a) direction, (b) extent, (c) force, (d) timing, and (e) tone; in relationship to equilibrium and movement (cerebellum for balance, locomotion, and learned skills for coordination)
TRS	Tracks (white fiber connections to various nuclei)
MLF	Medial longitudinal fasiculus
ANS	Autonomic nervous system

The following developmental phases, based upon Moore (Gilfoyle et al., 1990), reflect growth and development in the seven functional areas in relationship to the archi, paleo, and neo systems. The addition of the central pattern generator concept within each of the three functional systems enhances Moore's growth model, "Thus, movement patterns generated within the CNS or in response to external stimuli gradually become integrated into a smoothly coordinated system capable of interacting purposely with the environment..." (p. 54). From conception through maturity, the human organism grows within different contexts with changing object relationships. Intra- and inter-coordination of CPGs in the spinal cord, brain stem, forebrain, cortex, midbrain, and cerebellum have resulted in functional columnar arrangements to locate memory traces in the somatosensory and the visual cortex, along with localized centers to recognize specific attractor object relationships (face, voice, food [smell], touch, and vestibular/proprioceptive responses) from environmental input.

Therefore, archi, paleo, neo, and neo-neo-functional systems evolved to handle the complexity of occupational engagement in activities and relationships in changing environments, where CPGs

"...typically transform excitatory tonic driving input into detailed spatiotemporal patterns of oscillatory activity" (Yuste et al., 2005, p. 477). Grillner et al. (2005) described these functional systems as microcircuits that are oscillatory in nature, and integrative, depending upon the tasks of the individual. As noted by Bronfenbrenner (1979), the ecology within human development exerts a multidimensional impact. The spatiotemporal adaptation of the rhythmical and oscillatory central pattern generation throughout the nervous system provides a neuophysiological basis for sensorimotor integration, object relationship responses, and the development of appropriate affect to meet physical and sociocultural occupational demands for environmental adaptation (Llorens, 1976). The following occupational physiology sequences, based upon Moore (1990, pp. 41 & 61), are depicted (for each system sequence noted, there is a continuum of temporality, with some subsystem components starting later than others). The central pattern generator locations were discussed and referenced previously. The following typology of the archi, paleo, neo and neo-neo systems is based upon MacLean, (1973), and Moore, from Gilfoyle et al. (2000).

Archi system developmental phases, structures, CPG locations, and behaviors:

1. Archi elemental components: 4–12 weeks gestational age–10 years. Rhythmical generation of (a) postural sequences and spontaneous movements, coordination (automatism), and olfactory discrimination; (b) breathing, sucking, and swallowing; (c) homeostasis and endocrine functions—autonomic nervous system; (d) asleep or awake, alert and attending; (e) beginning balance and spatiotemporal orientation.
2. The main structures of earliest myelination and function are the (a) basal ganglia (part of amygdala [olfaction], subthalamic nucleus, stantia nigra) (background movement patterns), (b) propriospinal tracts and medial longitudinal fasiculus (craniospinal sensory receptors [general and special] and effectors to muscles and glands (tonic system), tegmentum (central core of brainstem), (c) epithalamus, hypothalamus, (d) reticular (autonomic) systems, and (e) vestibulocerebellum (coordination system).
3. Central pattern generator locations: Spinal cord, brain stem, reticular activating system, hypothalamus.

4. Developmentally purposeful activity components: rooting, sucking, swallowing, visual searching, fixation, and tracking while the head and body are moving in space, balance and equilibrium, communication, occupational balance for growth, hormonal responses and daily rhythms (awake occupations, sleep, rest), and internal visceral environment.

Paleo system developmental phases, structures, CPG locations, and behaviors.

1. Paleo elemental components: 5 months gestational age–7 years: Rhythmical generation of (a) patterns of postural adaptations, (b) locomotion (direction, extent, force), (c) ballistic (fast) movements and protopathic responses, (d) motivation and memory circuits, (e) visceral, (f) emotional tone or 3 Fs (feeding, fighting, reproduction), and stability (safety, pleasure, contentment, spirituality vs. fear, anger, rage, violence [continuum]), and (g) visual, auditory, and somatsensory responses.
2. The paleo structures most responsible for these functions, respectively, are the (a) basal ganglia (globus pallidus) (background movement), (b) spinocerebellum (coordination system), (c) motor center of subthalamus (survival) and ventral pathways of spinal cord (protection), (d) the limbic lobe and insula (affective system) (cingulate gyrus, parahippocampal gyrus, and hippocampus, amygdala, septal area), and (e) midbrain tectum—colliculi.
3. Central pattern generator locations: basal ganglia, limbic system, cerebellum.
4. Developmentally purposeful activity components: learning about harmful sensations; postural adjustment of the head, in relationship to the body and the supporting surface; locomotion in all positions and stabilization for upright postures and hand-to-mouth activity; initiation and orientation of, and to, activity in space and time per occupational demands; and appropriate affective object-action sequences.

Neo and neo-neo system developmental phases, structures, CPG locations, and behaviors.

1. Neocortical elemental components (in concert with archi and paleo systems): 8 months gestational age-maturity. Rhythmical

generation of (a) exploration, (b) learned skills, (c) semi-automatic learned responses, (d) information integration, (e) perception and appreciation through discrimination, (f) plan, program, and execute skills and survival stratagems.

2. Neo-neocortical elemental components involve rhythmical generation of (a) self-reflexivity for judgment, (b) emotional stability, (c) motivation, (d) memory (circuits), (f) semantics and syntax.

3. The neo structures most responsible for these functions, respectively, are the (a) dorsal pathways, (b) neocerebellum, (c) basal ganglia—caudate nucleus and putamen, (d) dorsal thalamus, and (e) frontal, temporal, parietal, and occipital lobes.

4. The neo-neo structures most responsible for these functions are the prefrontal and anterior temporal lobes working in concert with the limbic system.

5. Central pattern generator locations: basal ganglia, limbic lobes, premotor and supplementary motor cortices.

6. Developmentally purposeful activity components: Exploration, appreciation, and anticipation needed for planning, enhanced pro-gravity, and voluntary skills needed for precision in eating, writing, object manipulation, grooming and hygiene, and construction of meaning.

The author recommends the inclusion of this section of *Occupational Physiology*, that is, *central pattern generation of archi, paleo and neo systems*, be incorporated in the application of updates to the Llorens' model. The occupational physiology of *Functional CPG Systems* results from the integration of sensory stimuli, as found in purposeful activity. The author next describes this sensory integrative aspect of purposeful activity, as an inherent feature of adaptive occupation.

Sensory Integration of Neurochaotic CPGs Within Functional Systems

Korn and Faure (2003) cited G. Laurent (p. 822) regarding the perceptual recognition and categorization involved in "...sensory networks...[which] should be viewed as a system ...our current thinking about sensory integration...is too often linear and passive: one should rather consider them as active and internal processes where a major role is devoted to the dynamic of the brain circuits themselves." The central nervous system uses sensory systems to activate representational neuronal assemblies in spatiotemporal patterns to encode and categorize data for storage and recall in addition to reducing distortion for optimal coherence.

Ayres (1960/1974) also described the role of sensory integration in neuronal assemblies, citing Hebb (p. 45): "to further explain the role of purposeful action in motor behavior..." Her remarks referred to the role of sensation in the temporal activation of a CPG "cell assembly." "A cell assembly repeatedly activated during a specific motor response will become associated with that response" (p. 45). This concept may further explain von Holst's magnet effect of the coupling together of automatisms critical for a given occupational demand. Ayres (1960/1974) noted that the cell assembly concept, as explained by Hebb, referred not only to how individuals learn, but that it may also explain the formation of readiness in neural structures for what has been learned and genetically retained through phylogeny and ontogeny. "...The patterning of motor responses are further examples. Perhaps these neurophysiological mechanisms were learned through cell assembly association with efferent activity and became embedded in the genetic structure. The essential point is that animals were engaged in purposeful activity that provided both the functional demand and the stimuli that became associated with it" (p. 45). The importance of innate behavior in reproduction, facilitated by the sensorimotor integration of CPG coupling in psychosexual development, supports Freud's assertion about the importance of rhythmical pattern generation in regard to object relations, affective development, and erogenous zone maturation.

According to Kandel et al. (1995), meeting functional demands means ensuring bodily homeostasis, which is very important in lieu of changing environmental conditions. Associative learning helps animals and people to correlate causal events in the environment with a predictable sensory cue. "In other words, the brain seems to have evolved to detect causal relationships in the environment as evidenced in correlated or associated events" (p. 661). This associative ability is instinctively important for reproduction; "Among innate behavior, we first consider sexual behavior" (Kandel et al., 1995, p. 553). Varied novel situations compel the learning of complex relationships to cope with instinctual needs.

A Systems Control Model to Explain the Inherent Value of Occupation

Occupational theory predicts that intrinsic and extrinsic motivation to meet homeostatic activity demands, including tissue needs, circadian rhythms, and innate drives, requires the occupational association and anticipation of causal or predictive activity relationships (Llorens, 1984a, 1984b). In fact, Llorens found an 80% agreement among various standardized factors in participants' conscious detection and differentiation of occupation components when requested to self-report upon their activity analysis feedback (Llorens, 1986, 1993). Intrapersonal activity analysis, conscious and unconscious, is a homeostatic process allowing for adaptation. To this end, Kendal et al. (1995) noted that "The impressive perceptual, cognitive, and emotional [archi, neo, and paleo system] capacities of the human brain would be of little value if the brain could not use them to organize behavior ... [which] integrates sensory and motor information into purposeful action" (p. 529).

Control system models can illustrate how a system maintains its occupational balance through intrinsic and extrinsic motivation, when certain occupational components needed for performance fall below specific set-point levels. This author's creation of Figure 9 is based upon Llorens' *science of occupational theory* construct (Llorens, 1984b), regarding the inherent need to search for, find, and integrate activity components (Section 1 of her theory; Llorens, 1970), for occupational enablement of occupational roles and behaviors (Section 3 of her theory; Llorens, 1991). According to Hebbs theory, as cited by Arshavsky (2003), Ayres, (1960/1974), and Kandel et al. (1995), cell assembly groups that are wired together for central pattern generation of purposeful activity are comprised of pertinent activity components as integrated archi, paleo, and neo (including neo-neo) occupational physiologic systems.

For example, the various growth model activity components in Section 1 (Llorens, 1970) act in concert as integrated (functional CPG) sensorimotor systems during occupational performance. These activity components provide the set-point signal (as means). Inherent motivational feedback detectors analyze occupational activities, tasks, and interpersonal relationships in Section 3 (as ends). When the balance for occupational association of activity components (enablers) fall below needed role performance levels in Section 3,

FIGURE 9. Occupational Theory: A Systems Control Model Explains the Inherent Value of Activity. From Kandel et al. (1995) (Reproduced and Adapted with Permission). Intrinsic and Extrinsic Motivation is Postulated to Explain the Inherent Value of Activities, Occupations, Tasks, and Relationships, as a Measure of the Variability in Occupational Adaptedness

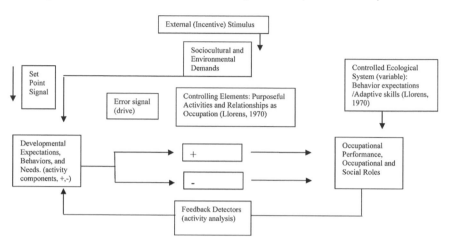

set-point activity component levels determine and choose/select the needed predicted/causal purposeful activities and relationships (Section 2; Llorens, 1970). The controlling elements (purposeful activities and relationships [including occupational readiness and environment modification activities]) to maintain occupational homeostasis are chosen/selected from occupational forms and interpersonal relationships in the physical and sociocultural environmental milieu. The occupational therapy process follows this same logic through activity analysis of the person components (occupational enablement), their associated occupations, and their environmental context (Llorens, 1966, 1967a, 1970, 1971, 1972, 1973, 1975, 1976, 1991, 1997a; Llorens & Adams, 1978; Llorens & Bernstein, 1963; Llorens & Donaldson, 1983; Llorens & Johnson, 1966; Llorens, Levy, & Rubin, 1964; Llorens & Rubin, 1962, 1967; Llorens, Rubin, Braun, Beck, & Beall, 1969; Llorens et al., 1964; Llorens & Shuster, 1977; Llorens & Young, 1960).

This control system model illustrates how a system maintains its occupational balance through intrinsic and extrinsic motivation when certain occupational components needed for performance fall below specific set-point levels.

Occupational Theory in the NICU

Infant and Family Vulnerability

According to Moore (Gilfoyle et al., 1990), CNS vulnerability and damage within the seven structural areas of the CNS, previously described, could occur as a result of many factors, including hypoxic-ischemic trauma and infection. Specific focal areas of damage might occur not only in the more vulnerable, newer structural areas, and where there are large metabolic costs and nerve cell pattern generation systems, but also to nerve cell pathway tracts and cell bodies in the white matter. In addition, trauma in or to the vascular system can create a lack of oxygen for these areas. The small capillaries in the watershed areas, where two different blood supply areas end and begin, are also areas of increased vulnerability.

Infant Occupational Physiology

In the NICU, infants are at risk for maladaptive growth and development in the central pattern generator cellular mechanisms and structures located in the archi, paleo, and neo systems. Ideally, brain stem pattern generation for breathing, sucking, swallowing, and heart rate is synchronous. However, pre-term infants frequently exhibit difficulty in the coordination of these functions (Bazyk, 1990). Studies of hypoxia in mammals indicate that damage to the brain stem CPG profoundly affects this synchronization (Akay, Lipping, Moodie, & Hoopes, 2002). Modulatory influences on the brain stem might have a similar effect. Motorically, infants use postural rhythms and movements to adapt (self-regulate) through sensory integration to their environment and to provide social interactive cues to caregivers through postural adjustments (Als, 1989). Therefore, insult or injury to the cortical, mid brain, cerebellar, brain stem, or spinal pattern generators may affect the CPG coupling, thereby inhibiting the assimilation of sensory information for coordination of movement sequences (Dubbeldam, 2001; Ferrari et al., 2002; Prechtl, 2001). Additionally, infants normally establish synchronous awake and alert states (Prechtl & Nolte, 1984), as sleep wake cycles are a function of cortical pattern generators that establish physiological states of alertness (Kuhle et al., 2001). The occupational physiology of self-regulation, state liability, and alertness are posited to correlate with central pattern generation in attention and arousal (Lydic, 1989) and for physiological homeostatic needs, all of which can be impacted by hypoxia (Gilfoyle et al., 1990). In summary, inefficient sensorimotor integration of CPGs affects the mutuality or coupling, albeit *magnet effect* described by von Holst (1973) in the totality or *relative coordination* as "a type of neural cooperation" (p. 29) to allow "switching" from one mode of occupation to another.

Family Occupational Physiology

Parenting is usually associated with reciprocity and mutuality (Bronfenbrenner, 1979). However, the parents of an NICU infant are forced to cope with a situation that challenges their self-efficacy beliefs (Hess et al., 2004). Parents oftentimes experience shock over their infant's circumstances (Dudek-Shriber, 2004), which creates stress and disrupts homeostatic central pattern generation (Wright, 2004), possibly resulting in physical fatigue or disorientation. The limbic system, an important central pattern generator for the psychosocial aspects of occupational enablement could be impacted (Gilfoyle et al., 1990), and emotions may be difficult to control from a psychodynamic perspective. In general, the parents of a high-risk infant may be in shock and find they have shifted from comfort and enjoyment to the pattern generation of survival-based needs.

Influencing Occupational Physiology in the NICU through Purposeful Activity

Occupational Enablement and Performance Behavior

The expanded Llorens model provides a theoretical basis to achieve growth and development through purposeful activities and relationships which "stimulate, facilitate, inhibit, and motivate" (Llorens, 1991, p. 50) intra- and inter-coordination of central pattern generation as means (Section 1; enablement of *Developmental Expectations, ehaviors, and Needs*) and ends (time use/roles in *Behavior Expectations and Adaptive Skills*). Llorens' thesis statement maintains:

That occupational therapy is a facilitation process which assists the individual in achieving mastery of life tasks and the ability to cope as efficiently as possible with the life expectations made of him [or her] through the mechanisms of selected input stimuli and availability of practice in a suitable environment (Llorens, 1970, p. 93).

Occupational screening and assessment in the NICU focuses upon the infant's interactive process for social interactions and participation in relationships, motoric processes, state control and alertness, physiological response to stress, and feeding abilities (American Occupational Therapy Association, 2006, 2007), all of which can be found (in general terms) in Sections 1 and 3 of Llorens' schematic (as function to dysfunction continuums). The occupational therapist considers both infant and family occupational enablement and occupational performance roles and time usage involved in play/leisure, work/learning, self-care, and rest/relaxation contexts.

Occupation: Purposeful Activities and Relationships in the NICU

Occupational therapy practice in the NICU is an example of how occupational therapists use occupation (Section 2 of Llorens' schematic; postulates regarding change) as a medium to promote the basic regulatory activities of the neonate. In addition to specific occupational readiness activities for feeding and movement and environmental modification activities for positioning and stress reduction, the occupational therapists must also consider the infant within the caregiver and family system to enhance optimal social interactions and movement organization. This perspective entails promoting the NICU infant's learning, play, restfulness, and caregiver interaction occupational performance.

Areas targeted for support are infant neurobehavioral and physiological development and consultation with nursery staff about infant positioning, feeding, and handling. Also, the occupational therapist establishes educational objectives for parent self-efficacy (Hess et al., 2004) to learn infant feeding techniques, infant awake/sleep cycles, cues for social interaction and coping, infant development, and positioning (Caretto, Topolski, Linkous, Lowman, & Murphy, 2000; Olson & Baltman, 1995; Whitley & Cowan, 1991). The next section describes the occupational physiology of the homeostatic control mechanism (Figure 10) for activities and relationships in the NICU.

FIGURE 10. Occupational Physiology of Activity Using a Sensory Integration Processing Model. The Sensory Processing of Purposeful Activi ies, Environments, and Relationships as Causal Agents in the Mediation of Occupational Physiology for Adaptive Spatiotemporal and Occupational Adaptation. Adapted and Reproduced with Permission from Llorens (1991), and Johansson (1998), also see Silberzahn (1978) (see Appendix A)

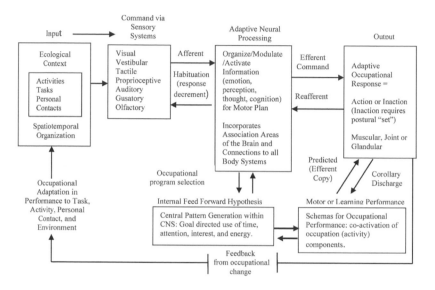

As shown in Figure 10, specialized sensory receptors provide information to the brain from a command via the sensory systems. Afferent information is tempered for adaptive neural processing, and occupational programs are then selected through internal feed forward patterns that are generated for goal-directed behaviors. These patterns reflect motor or learning performance schemas and provide a predicted response that is adjusted for the specific occupational demand, thereby generating an adaptive occupational response.

Sensory integration and sensorimotor processing reflect the influence of occupational activities on life task performance. And the role of activities and relationships are embedded within the ecological context in which they occur (Llorens, 1991). The occupational physiology of CPG theories endorses the importance of sensory systems in the shaping of the CPG cellular and synaptic structural interactions for environmental entrainment. The control system model (Figure 9) illustrates how activities are inherently associated with contexts and purpose and then recorded in memory for consolidation and retrieval (Arshavsky, 2003; Kandel, 2006) in the homeostatic balance of developmentally appropriate affective object relations (Freud, 1938; Graybiel, 1997; Hall, 1954; Llorens, 1976). As noted in Figure 10, the sensory processing for this homeostatic process considers use of purposeful activities, environments, and relationships as causal agents in the mediation of occupational CPG physiology for spatiotemporal and occupational adaptation.

Activity theory posits that the components of an activity produce an output greater than the sum of their composite parts (Llorens, 1986, 1993). As noted in Figure 10, afferent feedback to the CPG networks, through corollary discharge, adjusts the accuracy of intended (predicted) movements (von Holst, 1973). According to Prochazka (1993), "... the most important attribute of animal motor control systems is the ability to anticipate and adapt" (p. 13). Llorens (1986) called the ability to anticipate a "performance expectation" (p. 104). Pearson (2000) concluded that "An attractive concept is that persistent errors in behavior are detected by proprioceptors, and these error signals recalibrate the magnitude of feedforward signals" (p. 743).

The growth models contained in *Facilitating Growth and Development* provide a continuum of function and dysfunction against which to measure change. Facilitating activities and relationships provides the medium for adaptation in the NICU environment.

Neuroplasticity Through Occupation

Pearson (2000) noted that a method of intervention that quickly influences how the CPGs will initiate new patterns of rhythmical behaviors is through task modification. Modifying a task provides a new "set" of behavior expectations for specific task demands (social-emotional, cognitive, perceptual, and motor). These strategies have been repeatedly cited by Llorens (1966, 1967b, 1968, 1971, 1972, 1973, 1975, 1984a, 1986, 1993, 1999; Llorens & Adams, 1978; Llorens & Bernstein, 1963; Llorens & Johnson, 1966; Llorens, Levy, & Rubin, 1964; Llorens & Rubin, 1962, 1967; Llorens et al., 1964, 1969; Llorens & Young, 1960). In this respect, a slower neurological adaptation can occur as a result of sustained sensory bombardment as the sensitization, association, or habituation involved in training and practice. The integrative actions of the CPGs provide a living system with the capacity and capability for environmental adaptation through selected activity and affective object relationships. These tenants hold true for infants and their families in the NICU, where spatiotemporal and occupational adaptation include processes such as the sprouting of new neurological connections and redistribution of nerve cell body genetic material in response to specific sensory input, and where sensory motor movement reactivation enhances synaptic strengthening.

Pearson (2000) noted that the flexibility of the CNS to adapt to change (new learning or refinement of previously learned behaviors) and to reestablish purposeful movements after CNS injury is dependent upon two processes.

> The first is the ability of the nervous system to precisely regulate complex patterns of activity in numerous muscles according to the demands of the task and the mechanics of the motor system. The second [process] is the capacity of pattern-generating networks to adapt slowly in response to persistent changes in use, modifications of elements within the system, and maintained alterations in external conditions (p. 723).

According to Pearson (2000), one element in the neurophysiology of pattern phase cycles has to do with coupling (excitatory or inhibitory) in the degrees of movement needed for a specific task, in addition to the environmental demands and socio-emotional context. As previously noted, neuromodulation and the alternation in the oscillatory pacemaker bursts, or neuron coupling, is posited to explain the CPG mechanism (Arshavsky, 2003; Kuo, 2002; Marder & Bucher, 2001; Pearson, 2000).

The capacity for adaptive changes within and between the CPG systems may occur as short-term or long-term changes. Short-term adaptation is dependent upon the intensity and timing of activity patterns, whose afferent input in turn regulates the independent bodily action sequences needed for the task. In long-term adaptation, afferent input plays a major role in either positive or negative system change. Either lack of afferent input or non-rewarding habitual afferent input results in weaker afferent coupling between CPG neurons and less excitatory influence on the CPG itself (probably due to poor coupling).

Maintaining the motor elements for the appropriate mechanics of task completion requires the afferent cueing for the parameters of the task, which modifies pattern generating networks. Therefore, it is highly likely that long-term changes in the commands from the coordinated effects of the CPGs to motor neurons result from afferent signals that have been significantly and persistently altered (Pearson, 2000).

Discussion

Neural plasticity occurs through the inherent value and afferent reinforcement found in activities, tasks, and relationships, all of which occur within specific contexts that permit participation (Llorens, 1991, 1999; Pearson, 2000). This relationship is shown in Figure 9 as a homeostatic control model, with the sensory processing needed for internal activity analysis and occupation intervention elaborated upon in Figure 10. In the NICU, occupational therapy intervention is selected upon the basis of infant and family *Developmental Expectations, Behaviors and Needs*, and *Behavior Expectations and Adaptive Skills* (Llorens, 1970). Sensory input affects CPG tonic discharge and phasic timing, frequency, and amplitude through the convergence of multiple sensory stimuli from associated task components. According to Pearson (2000), "The detailed structure of activity patterns in individual groups of motor neurons is . . . established by the pattern of afferent input from the body and limbs" (p. 731). That way, "combinations of feedback signals are acted upon . . . rather than 'hard-wired' private loops for each sensory modality" (Prochazka, 1993, p. 12). Moreover, cutaneous afferents were found to converge upon and reorganize the CPG function in spinalized neonatal rats due to weight bearing and tactile contact of the hind limbs with the supporting surface (Commissiong et al., 1991). Additionally, skin receptors are identified as the most important source of information for spatiotemporal adaptation. These findings support occupational therapy activities and relationships for infants, in addition to family learning from educational occupational tasks, resulting in anticipatory performance (Hess et al., 2004; Llorens, 1986).

"The extent of [CNS] recovery depends upon the site and the extent of injury, and on the rehabilitation procedures" (Pearson, 2000, p. 739). According to activity theory, occupational association and selection of occupational form from environmental attractors depends upon the occupational demands of task components and from the intrinsic and extrinsic motivation and reinforcement (internal and external) of the task. Occupational therapy intervention utilizes occupational activities and interpersonal relationships for occupational performance intervention "in a suitable environment" (Llorens, 1970, p. 93). Consideration of how the sensory factors of an activity or task influence occupational physiology in relative (switching) and absolute (superimposition) CPG coordination (Redgrave et al., 1999; von Holst, 1973) assists in the analysis of which activities, relationships, and contexts will facilitate the occupational change process (Johansson, 1998; Prochazka, 1993). This strategy is supported by Pearson's speculation about the change mechanism for adaptation. *"An interesting issue, therefore, is whether the mechanisms underlying functional recovery are related to those that are involved in the day to day maintenance of the system* [italics added]" (Pearson, 2000, p. 733). The author cited multiple neuroscientists whose research indicated that changes in CPGs can be measured by the frequency of spontaneous tonic activity in a single CPG neuron and through the strength of phasic bursts between coupling mechanisms. In cases of central nervous system damage, new strategies developed through "behavioral substitution" (Pearson, 2000, p. 738) occur when there is a markedly different generation of patterns, with sprouting of undamaged afferents due to selected sensory input, resulting in CPG neural plasticity.

Occupational change involves transitional phases in the rhythmical coupling needed for CPG switching (Arshavsky, 2003; Marder & Bucher, 2001; Redgrave et al., 1999; Wright, 2004) and superimposition (Cotterill, 2001; von Holst, 1973). This flexibility facilitates multidimensional interactions in cognitive, emotional/affective, psychodynamic, motor, and social neurobehavioral schema. As noted by Moore (Gilfoyle et al., 1990), the emergent and distributed nature of CPG integration in the archi, paleo, and neo systems occurs throughout development. Occupational physiology, as a sensory integrative process, entrains CPGs in the inherent value of activity for environment and organism mutuality and reciprocity (Llorens, 1984a). According to Kandel et al. (1995), in *"...place preference conditioning, ...* an animal learns to increase its contact with environments in which it has previously encountered positively reinforcing stimuli (sex, food, drink) and minimal contact with environments that are aversive or dangerous" (p. 610). Therefore, control system homeostatic mechanisms link an ecological context with recognized activities and relationships that are inherently survival serving.

Conclusion Part 2

Different developmental stages and times during the life cycle represent a qualitatively different human organism. According to Llorens (1970, 1976, 1991), developmental processes promote adaptive skills and behaviors or person occupation environment dynamic interactions. Furthermore, studies indicate that specific times throughout the developmental life cycle offer critical windows to activate adaptive human patterns and behaviors (Dunn & Brown, 1997; Oppenheim, 1984; Touwen, 1989). In regard to the theory and science of occupation (Llorens, 1984a), Ayres (1972) said that "The early developmental steps, determined by evolutionary history, have been "preprogrammed" into the brain at conception, but ontogenetic experience is necessary for the full expression of the inherent developmental tendencies" (Ayres, 1972, p. 4).

Llorens' conceptualization of (a) developmental behaviors, expectations, and needs, and (b) behavior expectations and adaptive skills (Llorens, 1970, 1976, 1991) supports person, occupation, and environmental mastery and competence through endogenous movements coupled with exogenous activities. Occupation in relevant contexts culminates in occupational performance activities, roles, and relationships for sociocultural and environmental adaptation. Current research into the theory of central pattern generators adds coherence and credence to the concept of neuroplasticity through occupational physiology, where developmental phases offer critical windows for specific aspects of growth and development.

PART 3: APPLICATION OF NEW CONCEPTS AND NEURO-PSYCHOLOGICAL ELEMENTS

This section focuses upon the application of the recommended changes to the Llorens model from Parts 1 and 2, in addition to a continued focus on activity theory and application of health models in the promotion of wellness and prevention of disability. The changes to Llorens' model expand the theoretical framework and premises of *Facilitating Growth and Development* to provide a new theoretical framework.

Revisions, Modifications, and Additions to the Llorens Model

Revision to Llorens' psychodynamic expectations, behaviors, and needs expands affective object relations in *erogenous zone* development. Furthermore, the psychodynamic activity component was modified to link the development of *moral character activities* and *relationships* with psychosexual phases of development. The author also modified the sensorimotor activity component to include *occupational physiology*, which explains the role of central pattern generation in the intrinsic adaptive value of activities and relationships. New activity components added to Llorens' theory are *Social Learning Theory*, which explains how observed behaviors become cognitively regulated through self-efficacious performance of activity. Also, a *Bioeceological Model* explains the importance and impact of activity contexts, and *Discovery Learning* expands Piaget's theory regarding the role of activity in the development of creative problem-solving. The applied changes are represented in Table 5. Additionally, Appendix B illustrates the author's additions to the original schematic (shown in italics), along with any deletions to Llorens' most recently updated (1991) model.

Last, the author provides a comparison of the expanded Developmental Theory of Occupational Therapy with other health models, in addition to providing a data collection tool that reflects the model's constructs. Finally, NICU practice and process models provide an illustration of these components. A case illustration emphasizes these practical solutions in practice.

La Corte Expansion to Llorens Model

Changes Applied to Section 1: Developmental Expectations, Behaviors, and Needs

In Section 1 the author expanded the sensorimotor occupation component to include *occupational physiology*. This expansion describes intrinsic central pattern generator factors as functional systems in the "mental operations that originate from sensory motor acts carried out as external actions with external objects [that] are involved in task, activity, and occupation component use" (Llorens, 1986, p. 104). The concept of occupational physiology is

TABLE 5. Schematic Representation of Achieving Growth and Development

Section I – Part 1
Developmental Expectations, Behaviors and Needs (Occupational Enablement)

Sensorimotor		Physical-Motor (Gesell)	Psychosocial (Erikson)	Psychodynamic	
Neuropsychological (Ayres)	Occupational Physiology (Moore, van Holst)			Psychosexual — Object-Affect-Action Erogenous Zone Development (Freud) (as discussed by Freud/Grant/Hall)	Character Development (Peck/Havighurst)
0-2 yrs. Sensorimotor / Tactile, vestibular, visual, auditory, olfactory, gustatory functions	Central Pattern Generator: Archi System; 7wks GA-10 yrs: Homeostatic, circadian rhythms, endocrine func/, attention; orientation time/ space; spontan. movements	0-2 yrs. / Head sags / Fisting / Gross motion / Walking / Climbing	Basic Trust vs. Mistrust/Oral / Sensory / Ease of feeding / Depth of sleep / Relax of bowels	0-4 yrs. Oral Zone: Dependency; Init. Aggress; Object cathexes with breast/bottle, thumb/pacifier; Genital erogenous zone arousal and autoerotism.	Infancy: Amoral Type / Follows whims and impulses; Self-gratifying; Lacks internal moral prin. conscious, or superego.
6 mo.–4 yrs / Integration of Body Sides / Gross motor plan / Form & space Balance / Post. and bilateral integration / Body scheme-develop	Central Pattern Generator: Paleo System: 5 mes. GA-7 yrs / Emot. reg. + balance; patterns of locomotion; affective responses; orientation vis., auc, somatosensory; protection	2-3 yrs. / Runs / Balances / Hand preference / Coordination	Autonomy vs. Shame & Doubt/ Muscular-Anal / Conflict between holding on & letting go	0-4 yrs. Anal-Sadistic Zone: Autoerotism incr. with sphincter control; Independence; Resistiveness; Self-assertiveness; Narcissism; Ambivalence; Genital masturbation is cyclic and oscillating, intersperse; with latency; Eyes: visual expl, "looking" discrimination.	→
3-7 / Discrimination / Refined tactile, kinesth, visual, auditory, olfact. gustatory functions	Central Pattern Generator: Neocortical System: 8 mos. GA-maturity: Exploratory/ discrim, skillful,, info. in.eg, creative/art,, moto / planning/ semi-auromatic rnvts.	3-6 yrs. / Coordination more graceful / Muscles develop / Skills develop	Initiative vs. Guilt/ / Locomotor-Genital / Aggressiveness / Manipulation / Coercion	3-6 yrs. Phallic Zone: (oedipal object relations) / Social expression, pivotal in cha:: development; Deep affection opposite sex parent; Auth. struggle/identification same sex parent; Genital masturbation, anal sphincter control; Eyes: visual exploration; looking" at playmates and adult (parents) genitalia, observation of toileting Knowledge sublimation for investigation.	Early Childhood: / Expedient type: / Self Centered, conscience and superego not consistently rational; needs external controls to guide behavior.
Abstract Thinking / Conceptualization / Complex relations / Read, write numbers	Central Pattern Generator / Neo-Neo System; Birth- / maturity: self reflect/judgment / emotional stability; motivation; / memory circuits; semantics	6-11 yrs. / Energy dev / Skill practice to attain proficiency	Industry vs. Inferiority/ / Latency / Wins recognition / thru productivity / Learns skills & tools	6-13 yrs. Latency or Partial Latency due to sexual inhibition; / Initiation of mastery of skills, strong defenses. Genital masturbation may be suppressed, or continue; Eyes identify object attractors; Init in mastery of skills; Strong defenses.	6-13 yrs. Either of these types: / Conforming: Rule bound behavior, consequences not relevant. Crude conscience / Irrational Conscientious: follows set of internalized ideals; rigid superego; disregards effects of actions on others.
Continue to develop / Conceptualization / Complex relations / Read, write numbers	Central Pattern Generation is neurochaotically emergent and distributive throughout Archi/Paleo/Neo and Neo-Neo systems for Occupational	11-13 yrs. / Rapid growth / Poor posture / Awkwardness	Identity vs. Role / Confusion/Puberty & Adolescence / Identification / Social Roles	13 yrs - Genital Zone Maturation / Ability for primacy, cont. masturbation; Breasts: (women) mature as erogenous zone and attractor. Eyes: Visual excitement of sexual objects (images, symbols); Emancipation from parents; Occup. Decisions; Role experiment; Re–cexam of values.	13- Rational – Altruistic: Uses judgment to guide interpersonal activities; Consideration of others as much as consideration of self. Ongoing dev. throughout life span.
Development presumably maintained	Performance (stimuli association, selection, process/engagement)	Growth established and maintained	Intimacy vs. Isolation / Young Adulthood / Commitments Body & ego mastery	Outgrow need for parent validation; identify with others, selection of love object, sexual aims, and sublimation of sexual energy for creativity.	Give and receive love, productive endeavors interpersonal endeavors (Adler & Jung, as discussed by Breger, 2000, Peck & Havighurst, 1960; Schellanburg, 1978)
Alterations begin to occur in sensory functions, conceptplzm., and memory	These dynamic systems work together; and exhibit variability in their complexity.	Alterations begin to occur in motor behavior, strength and endurance	Generativity vs. Stagnation / Adulthood; Guiding next ger:. / Creative, productive	Emotional responsibilities may lessen; Physical and econ. Independence; Accepted shift from survival to enjoyment.	
Alterations in sensory functions, conceptplzm, and memory		Alterations in motor behavior, strength and endurance	Ego Integrity vs. Despair/Maturity / Accept. life cycle	Continued growth after middle age; Inner trend toward survival.	

Ecology of the Microsystem (Bronfenbrenner, 1979). Provides dynamic opportunities for spatotemporal (ontogenetic) adaptation, or occupational enablement, in the meso, exo and macrosystem spheres of growth and development.

Note: Adapted and Reproduced with Permission. From Llorens (1991, p. 48-49). Provides dynamic opportunities for spatotemporal (ontogenetic) adaptation, or occupational enablement, in the meso, exo and macrosystem spheres of growth and development. Performance tasks and roles throughout the lifespan. In C. Christiansen and C. Baum, (Eds.,, Occupational therapy: Overcoming human performance deficits, (pp. 48-49). Thorofare, NJ: Charles B. Slack

TABLE 5. Continued

Section 1 – Part 2
Developmental Expectations, Behaviors and Needs
(Occupational Enablement)

Sociocultural (Gesell)	Social (Cognitive) Language		Activity of Daily Living (Gesell)
	Language (Gesell)	Social Cognition & Self-efficacy (Bandura)	
Oral erotic activity Individual: Mothering person most important Immediate family group important	Small sounds Coos Vocalizes, Listens Speaks	Infancy Observational Learning Perceptual consequences of actions-differentiation of self from others	Recognizes bottle Holds spoon Holds glass Controls bowel
Parallel play Often alone Recognizes extended family	Identifies objects verb. Asks "Why?" Short sentences	Early Childhood: Anticipatory behavior results from family, school and peer relationships	Feeds self Helps undress Recognizes simple tunes No longer wets at night
Seeks companionship Makes decisions Plays with other children Takes turns	Combines talking and eating Complete sentences Imaginative Dramatic		Laces shoes Cuts with scissors Toilets independently Helps set table
Group play and team activities Independence of adults Gang interests	Language major form of communication	7-12 yrs. Opportunities for creativity, Self rating of progress in meeting goals, Cognitive capacities challenged	Enjoys dressing up Learns value of money Responsible for grooming
Team games Organization important Interest in opposite sex	Verbal language predominates	Adolescence: Symbolic modeling by peers, teachers and parents results in Antecedent behavior	Interest in earning money
Group affiliation Family, social, civic interest	Non-verbal behavior used	Adulthood Occupational choice is determined by self-efficacy beliefs. Innovative planning for family and vocational adjustment	Concern for personal Grooming, mate, family
		Advancing Age: Re-evaluate efficacy for physical and productive activities Activity to maintain health efficacy	Accepting and adjusting to changes of middle age
		Old Age Use cognition to compensate for increased frailty	Adjusting to changes after middle age

Note: Reproduced and Adapted with Permission. From Llorens (1991, p. 48–49). Performance tasks and roles throughout the lifespan. In C. Christiansen and C. Baum, (Eds.), *Occupational therapy: Overcoming human performance deficits*, (pp. 48-49). Thorofare, NJ: Charles B. Slack.

Ecology of the Microsystem (Bronfenbrenner, 1979). Provides dynamic opportunities for spatiotemporal (ontogenetic) adaptation, or occupational enablement, in the meso, exo and macrosystem spheres of growth and development.

TABLE 5. Continued

Section 2
Achieving Activities and Relationships (Selected)
(Occupation for Performance in Work/Education, Play/Leisure, Self-care, and Rest/Relaxation Time Activities)

Integrative Sensorimotor Activities (Activation, organization, and modulation of all central processing/patterning to all body systems)	Developmental Activities (Play and learning occupations; skill achievement)	Symbolic Activities	Daily Life Tasks (All occupationally vital life tasks; performance in instrumental and daily care [maintenance] activities)	Interpersonal Activities
Focused Tactile, visual, auditory, olfactory, gustatory, vestibular and proprioceptive input	Dolls Animals Sand Water Excursions	Biting Chewing Eating Blowing Cuddling	Recognize food Hold feeding equipment Use feeding equipment	Individual interaction (Dyadic reciprocity according to Bronfenbrenner, 1979)
Physical positions and exercise, sucking, posturing, signaling comfort and distress. Body scheme and image, Postural-ocular control, Discrimination, Balancing, Motor planning	Pull toys Playground Clay Crayons Chalk	Throwing Dropping Messing Collecting Destroying	Feeding Toileting	Individual interaction Parallel play (Dyadic and N + 2 systems, according to Bronfenbrenner, 1979)
Listening Learning Skilled tasks & games	Being read to Coloring Drawing Painting	Destroying Exhibiting	Feeding Dressing Toileting Simple chores	Individual interaction Play small groups Dynamic group interaction and interdependency (Lewin, as described by Schellenburg, 1978)
Reading Writing Numbers	Scooters Wagons Collections Puppets Building (sand castles, block designs, tent houses)	Controlling Mastery	Feeding Dressing Grooming Spending	Individual interaction Groups Teams Clubs
All of the above available to be recycled	Weaving Machinery tasks Carving Modeling	All of the above available to be recycled	Feeding Dressing Grooming Pre-voc. skills	Individual interaction Groups Teams
	Arts Crafts Sports Club & interest groups Occupational Roles: Leisure Education Work	Purposeful Activities and Dyadic Reciprocity include sensorimotor integration, development of appropriate affective responses, and the ability to relate appropriately to objects (Llorens, p. 37)	Feeding Dressing Grooming Occupational Life role skills (ADL. & IADL.) Intuition Creativity Insight	Individual interaction Groups
	Developmental Mastery for Occupational Enablement	Mesosystem linkages to all other Micro, Exo, and Macro systems. (Bronfenbrenner, 1979)	Developmental Mastery for Successful Occupational Role Adaptation	

Note: Reproduced and Adapted with Permission. From Llorens (1991, p. 48-49). Performance tasks and roles throughout the lifespan. In C. Christiansen and C. Baum. (Eds.), *Occupational therapy: Overcoming human performance deficits*, (pp. 48-49). Thorofare, NJ: Charles B. Slack

87

TABLE 5. Continued

Section 3
Behavior Expectations and Adaptive Skills
(Environmental [physical and socio-cultural] Adaptation)

Developmental Tasks (Havighurst, Peck & Havighurst)	Human Ecology (Bronfenbrenner)	Ego-Adaptive Skills (Mosey; Pearce & Newton)	Discovery Learning through Play and Scaffolding (Bruner)	Intellectual Development (Piaget)
Learning to walk, talk, take solids Elimination	Differentiated perception and response; Dyadic change, visual disc. for shapes, mother's voice.	Ability to respond to mothering Mastering of gross motor responses	0-3 yrs: Enactive Stage, Motor learning of action sequences	Motor skills Integrated
Sex difference Form concepts of social and physical reality Relate emotionally to others Right vs. wrong Develop a conscience	Directing and controlling one's own behavior; Enjoys peek-a-boo, cuddling, looking at books, music, saying "no"	Ability to respond to routines of daily living Mastery of 3 dimensional space Sense of body image	→	Investigative Imitative Egocentric
Symbolic expressions of spirituality; Motivational quest for life's meaning	Coping successfully under stress: Ecological transitions between Microsystems, generalize objects and relationships to adapt to new contexts.	Ability to respond to routines of daily living Mastery of 3 dimensional space Tolerate frustrations Sit still Delay gratification	3-8 yrs: Iconic Stage. Visual memory for concrete objects and relationships stored in categorical schemas	Egocentrism reduced, Social increased Language to Represent Motor Behavior
Learn physical skills Getting along Reading, writing Values Social attitudes	Acquiring knowledge and skill; didactic activities of the occupational role entail new object relationships	Ability to perceive, sort, organize & utilize stimuli Work in groups	6-8 yrs.- developing through adulthood: Symbolic Stage Increasingly more diffuse ability for self consciousness reflectiveness	Orders experience Relates parts to wholes Deduction
More mature relationships Social roles Select occupation Achieving emotional independence	Establishing and maintaining mutually rewarding relationships: N=2 systems	Ability to accept & discharge responsibility Capacity for love		Systematic approach to problems Sense of equality Induction
Selecting a mate Starting a family, marriage, home Congenial social group	Modifying and constructing one's own physical, social, and symbolic environment: "power" connections shape policy, funding, politics, and philosophy of culture and sub-culture.	Ability to function independence Control drives Plan & execute Purposeful motions Obtain org. & use knowledge Participate in primary group Participate in variety of relationships Experiences self as acceptable Participate in mutually satisfying heterosexual relations		Development established and maintained
Civic & social responsibility Economic standard of living Development adult leisure activities Adjust to aging parents Adjust to decreasing physical health, retirement, death Age group affiliations - Meeting social obligations Occupational Self - themes of meaning (Jackson, Llorens)			Narrative (Bruner)	Alterations in other areas may affect

Ecology of the Exosystem (Bronfenbrenner, 1979) = Occ. (Role) Adaptation: the process of mutual accommodation between the person, their occupational activity, and the changing environment. Incorp. Occupational Readiness (Schultz & Schade, 1992a, 1992b).

Ecology of the Macrosystem = Prototype of culture and subculture (Bronfenbrenner, 1979); Includes occupational (a) forms (objects), (Nelson, 1986) (b) socialization (Mead, as discussed by Schellenburg, 1978), and, (c) performance. (Llorens, 1976) and, (d) context (Bronfenbrenner, 1979)

Adapted and Reproduced with Permission. From: Llorens (1991, p. 48-49). Performance tasks and roles throughout the lifespan. In C. Christiansen and C. Baum, (Eds.), *Occupational therapy: Overcoming human performance deficits*. (pp. 48-49). Thorofare, NJ: Charles B. Slack in keeping with the tenets of activity theory. Llorens (1986) cited Leont'ev (p. 105) to note the relationship between systemic formations of emergent and distributive mediational activity properties involving "psychophysiological/neurobehavioral mechanisms that reflect the transition between objective activity and function" (p. 105).

The psychodynamic occupation component in Section 1 offers a differing perspective about Freud's psychosexual theory than originally provided by Llorens. As noted in Table 3, Freud's hypothesis about the physiological aspect of erogenous zone development brings new light to the association of CPG rhythmical impulses for awareness, attention, and corresponding psychosocial object relations and development of affect. Through ontogeny, these survival-serving affective task properties became inherently embedded in the occupational physiology. Social experiences sensorially facilitate the psychosexual growth process. Corresponding to Freud's psychosexual development, the author used the Peck and Havighurst (1960) study to further expand the psychodynamics column. This expansion consists of the development of moral character illustrated in Table 5 of Section 1. Interestingly, Havighurst (1972) data for *Developmental Tasks* (Section 3 of Llorens' model) resulted from the Peck and Havighurst (1960) character development study (Peck and Havighurst, 1960, p. 156).

Albert Bandura's *social learning theory* and *self-efficacy beliefs* provide further expansion in the social language occupation component for Section 1. The developmental phases of Bandura's concepts fit nicely into Llorens' model as social *cognitive* language because of his emphasis on receptive language development in observational learning, self-regulation, and performance expectations.

Yuri Bronfenbrenner's *human ecology* framework correlates with Llorens' thesis statement and explains activities, relationships, and roles of the *microsystem, mesosystem, exosystem*, and the *macrosystem*, thereby expanding the context for activity during development. The microsystem is considered the major context for Section 1, while the exosystem and macrosystem are considered major contexts for Section 3. The mesosystem functions as the linkage between these systems, as physical, psychosocial, and cognitive ecological factors represented in Section 2. Thus, the mesosystem serves as a connector, catalyst, and reinforcer between occupational enablement and occupational role behavior.

Changes Applied to Section 2: Facilitating Activities and Relationships

As noted in Table 5, further explanation of *sensorimotor* activities for the purpose of assessment and intervention, adds more clarity to the mediational role of the sensory systems in the occupational physiology (activation, organization, and modulation) of central pattern generation as a basis for developmental mastery and adaptation. Additional descriptors include more behavioral items whose expression is dependent upon this sensorimotor integration between occupational physiology and neuropsychology, as noted in Section 1.

The overall emphasis of Section 2 hinges upon additional factors, such as *developmental activities* for object relations, where Llorens had noted the importance of play, learning occupations, and skill achievement in her discussion of this column in 1976 (p. 41). However, she omitted play from *developmental activities* in 1976. This author added play, learning occupations, and skill achievement in parenthesis for further clarification, in addition to *occupational roles* at the end of the *developmental activities* column, under which *leisure* was added to education and work. Occupational behaviors in these areas serve as a culmination of play, learning occupations, and skill achievement. Csikszentmihalyi (1997) described the relationship between play and later adaptive occupational role development as *finding flow*. The general nature of Section 2 as a mesosystem linkage to occupational enablement and occupational behavior role development appears centered in the middle bottom of the chart.

Llorens articulated *daily life tasks* as originating out of basic needs, such as feeding, grooming, self-care, and prevocational self-mastery. This author emphasized the importance of these daily life skills *as occupationally vital life tasks*, expanding this concept to mean both instrumental and daily maintenance activities and culminating in *occupational life role skills*, where habits, routines, and self-patterns establish *intuition, creativity*, and *insight* of self, family, and community.

Additions to the interpersonal activities column relate opportunities for affective and object relations to development. Bronfenbrenner's (1979) delineation of *dyadic reciprocity* and *dyadic and N + 2 systems*, also Kurt Lewin's (Schellenburg, 1978) historical theoretical premise of *dynamic group interaction and interdependency* through sensitivity training, helps to articulate how meaningful activities and relationships enhance affect and object relations.

Changes Applied to Section 3: Behavior Expectation and Adaptive Skills

Section 3 portrays how individuals apply their occupational enablement from Section 1 in various physical and sociocultural environments to meet occupational demands (behavior expectations) for skill mastery and adaptation. In the broad area of *developmental tasks* by Havighurst (1972), this author added Peck and Havighurst's (1960) discovery in their study of the psychology of character development that *symbolic expressions of spirituality* and a *motivational quest for life's meaning* were related to an inner need to believe in something greater than the self system, as an interconnectedness among all life. Llorens, in her manuscript *A Fifty-Five Year Odyssey of Body, Mind, and Spirit* (Llorens, 2004) cited Jackson and noted that "... global themes of meaning may guide the manner in which occupations are chosen and performed" (p. 9). The author's conclusion is that these themes of meaning, garnered from the experiences of doing, result in the *occupational self*.

Although Bronfenbrenner's theory of human ecology is integrated throughout this model to denote the diverse ecological spheres where activities and roles occur, *human ecology*, as *adaptive behavioral outcomes* are included as a separate category. Additionally, Bruner's work fits best with the task-oriented, role-bound growth phases of Section 3. Bruner's later emphasis upon *narrative* (Bruner, 1999) compliments the depiction of the *occupational self*. As noted in the changes applied to Section 1, the ecology of Bronfenbrenner's (1979) *exosystem* and *macrosystem* in Section 3 provides a systematic description for the observation and measurement of occupational role and occupational prototypes, as influenced by multiple activity factors.

Summary of Schematic Expansion

In closing, modifications, revisions, and additions applied to Llorens' model reflect the occupational theory and science constructs detailed in the occupational physiology of central pattern generation. Efficient sensorimotor integration results in spatiotemporal and occupational adaptation. Multiple occupational demands require emotional stability and utilize the motivational aspects of purposeful activity for psychophysiological (psychosexual and motivational character) behavioral development.

Additionally, constructs were introduced that correlate the role of cognition in perception to self-efficacy performance expectations for enhanced self-regulation in health. Also, the role of the environment as a facilitator, or barrier to activities and roles was addressed, along with problem-based learning, intersubjectivity, and narrative analysis of one's story. Last, the author inserted explanatory occupational theory constructs based upon Llorens' 1976 and 1991 textual delineations to further define and clarify each section heading. Table 5, Sections 1, 2, and 3, were adapted from Llorens (1991, pp. 48–49) (See Table 5).

Achieving Growth and Development: Correlation with Health Models

Activity Theory in Health

The emphasis of activity and participation in health by the World Health Organization's (WHO) International Classification of Functioning (ICF) (World Health Organization, 2001) further compliments *The Expanded Developmental Theory of Occupational Therapy*. WHO's activity-centered model (Figure 11) provides a basis to examine occupational performance in relationship to a person-occupation-environment interrelationship.

The author contrasts the WHO *Activity Model* with Llorens' expanded model, where Section 1 of *Achieving Growth and Development* corresponds to WHO's *Body Structures and Functions*, Section 2 with *Activities and Participation*, and Section 3 with *Contextual Factors* (see Table 6). Additionally, the author notes Baum and Law's (1997) model of *Occupational Performance* (Figure 12), and equates Sections 1, 2, and 3 of this model to a *Person-Occupation-Environment* (POE) construct for further comparison to Llorens' expanded schematic (see Table 6). In other words, the Baum and Law (1997) model purports a "PEO" construct. However, a different relationship is suggested here, with occupation as the connection between a person and their environment as POE. In the final part of this section on

FIGURE 11. Toward a Common Language for Functioning, Disability, and Health; ICF. From World Health Organization (2001). *Toward a Common Language for Functioning, Disability, and Health ICF*, p. 9. This Model Presents a Biopsychosocial Model that Focuses Upon the Individual their Occupational Activities and Participation within Relevant Contexts (reproduced with permission)

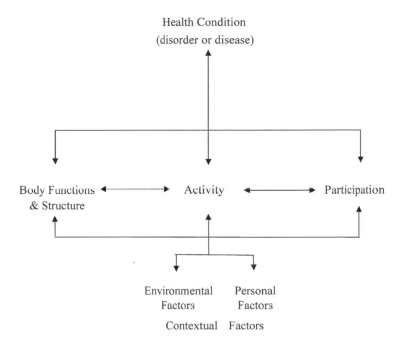

health perspectives, the author discusses mandates from the *Healthy Peoples* 2010 initiatives, *Conventions on the Rights of the Child*, and specific terminology from the *ICF* to support the theoretical basis for a NICU practice and process model.

Table 6 provides a comparison of the concepts discussed above.

Healthy Peoples, Conventions on the Rights of the Child, and the ICF

The *ICF* and *Person Occupation Environment* models portray the centrality of occupation to health. In the NICU, infants born

FIGURE 12. Baum and Law's (1997) Model of Occupational Performance. From Baum & Law (1997). These Authors Noted Model Adaptation
from Law et al. (1996) (reproduced with permission)

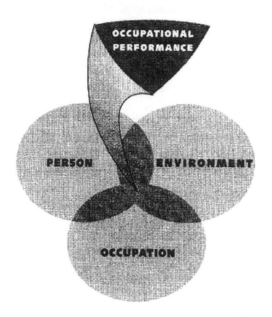

pre-term cannot participate in activities and relationships that support
typical growth and development. As previously noted, the leading cause of
cerebral palsy stems from preterm infants with low birth weight.
Secondary sequelae often accompany this motor disorder, ranging from
visual, hearing, and learning problems to mental retardation. The specific
goal for the Healthy People's Initiative, in respect to maternal and child
health objectives, is to decrease the percentage of cases of cerebral palsy
and learning impairments (United States Department of Health, Education,
and Welfare, 1980, 1990, 2001). In general, the Healthy People's Initiatives
aim to increase the quality and longevity of life and to decrease health
disparities in social justice (Kyler & Merryman, 2000).

    These initiatives focus upon outcomes pertaining to community
participation, a child's and family's mental health, social participation,
technology, and elimination of environmental barriers to daily life
activities. In essence, they focus upon the person, the person's
occupation, the environment, and health. Coinciding with the

TABLE 6. A Comparison of the Concepts in *Achieving Growth and Development* to the *WHO Activity Model*, the *Occupational Performance Model*, and the *Developmental Analysis, Evaluation, and Intervention Schedule*

Models	Major Concepts		
Achieving growth and development *Llorens expanded* (La Corte)	Developmental Needs, Behaviors, and Expectations (*Occupational Enablement*)	Facilitating Activities and Relationships (*Occupation for Performance in Work/Education, Play/Leisure, Self-Care, and Rest/Relaxation Time Activities*)	Behavior Expectations and Adaptive Skills (*Environmental [physical and socio-cultural] Adaptation*)
ICF (WHO)	Body Structures and Functions	Activities and Participation	Contextual (personal and environmental) Factors
Occupational performance model (Baum & Law, 1997) Modified as POE	Person	Occupation	Environment
Developmental analysis, evaluation, and intervention Schedule for infant and family occupations in the NICU (adapted from Llorens, 1977b)	Growth and development disruptions in daily activities relative to age, gender, life role, and condition for *Occupational Enablement (developmental needs, behaviors, and expectations)*	Occupational therapy activity and relationship plan for occupational *engagement and participation* (specific objectives keyed to problems list); Problem Identification in Areas of Occupational Performance Affected	Growth and development disruptions in daily activities relative to age, gender, life role, and condition in *Contextual Environmental Adaptation (socio-cultural and physical occupational behavior expectations and adaptive skills)*

Healthy People's Initiatives is the 2010 Express (Care Connection for Children, 2007). Maternal and Child Health (U.S. Department of Health and Human Services) collaborated with the American Academy of Pediatrics and other service organizations to develop the 2010 Express (Hanft, 2002). This initiative focuses upon child and family services, noting that families will partner with health care providers in decision-making for the services they receive, with monitoring of consumer satisfaction levels. Thus, national priorities, in addition to terminology in the ICF, philosophically denotes the importance of defining child and family participation as an outcome, and challenges occupational therapy's scope in developing occupation-based programs that focus upon the quality of life for children and their families. Moreover, an international document, *Convention on the Rights of the Child* (United Nations, 2002), provides that "Every child has the right to life, and States shall ensure, to the maximum, child survival and development" (p. 4). The next section identifies the *intersection* of theory, practice, and process.

Integrating Theory, Practice, and Process

Theoretical Premises and Concepts

Based upon (a) Llorens' original thesis statement (Llorens, 1970, p. 93 [see Part 1 of this issue]) and health care models described in Llorens (1997b) and AOTA (2001), (b) the theoretical schematic expansion introduced in Part 3 this issue, and (c) current concepts from international and national health initiatives, the author proposes the following adaptation of Llorens' premises (1970, pp. 93–94 [see Part 1 of this issue]).

1. That infant, parent, and family (person/family) *occupations* or *purposeful activities* are performed as tasks, activities, and relationships in a balanced and personally gratifying use of time in occupational performance tasks, activities, and relationships, known as education/work, play/leisure, basic and instrumental daily living (as self-care/maintenance), and rest/relaxation, and in life roles, routines, patterns, and habits.
2. Because of their inherent qualities of purposefulness and meaningfulness, occupations provide an *organizing* (*integrating*) *medium* to achieve growth and development across the lifespan.

3. That occupational physiology provides a basis for occupation.
4. That a person and their family develop simultaneously and chronologically as occupational beings in regard to *Developmental Expectations, Behaviors, and Needs* in the areas of neurophysiological-sensorimotor, physical-motor, psychosocial and psychodynamic abilities, and sociocultural, social cognitive language, and activities of daily living skills, which enable spatiotemporal adaptation of the person system.
5. That this need fulfillment promotes mastery and competence in these skills and abilities.
6. Consequently, person and/or family members exhibit *Behavior Expectations and Adaptive Skills* in the form of ego-adaptive and cognitive-intellectual skills, a range of developmental tasks, and relationships that are necessary to achieve satisfactory coping with life roles in the ecological contexts of the environmental system as occupational adaptation.
7. That the fundamental endowment of the person and the entrainment of the experiences received within the environment of the family come together to interact in such a way as to achieve positive early growth for both the person and family system.
8. That later environmental influence of extended family, community, social, and civic systems assist in the growth process.
9. That physical, occupational, and psychological trauma to the person or to family members related to disease, injury, environmental insufficiencies, or intrapersonal vulnerability can interrupt both the person and the family system's growth and developmental process.
10. That such growth interruption will cause a gap in the developmental cycle, resulting in a disparity between desired-expected person and family coping behavior and adaptive facility.
11. That assessment of the person and family *Behavior Expectations and Adaptive Skills* and *Developmental Expectations, Behaviors, and Needs* serve as indicators of occupational performance dysfunction and define specific occupational performance needs.
12. That occupational assessment is guided by the person and family system in the determination of needs for goal setting, whether for health promotion, disease prevention, modification of behavior, maintenance, habilitation, or rehabilitation.
13. That occupational therapy, through the skilled application of occupations, activities, tasks, and relationships, can link the person

and/or family and the environment system to purposeful activity (occupation) in regard to purposeful and meaningful time usage in areas of occupation (per #4) to achieve growth and development.

14. Additionally, that occupational therapy can assist in closing the gap between the person and/or family system and the environment system of desired expectation and ability and prevent or minimize the development of potential maladaptation related to insufficient nurturing or environmental barriers.

15. That the occupational therapy intervention process occurs through health promotion and disease prevention efforts on a one-to-one basis, in small and large groups, and through indirect learning experiences to achieve change in the desired directions. Multiple environments and options provide active person and/or family involvement in the occupational performance intervention process. (Adapted with permission from Llorens, 1970, pp. 93–94).

These premises summarize the expansion of Llorens' schematic, and pertinent health models as presented in Part 3 of this issue. They provide further support for her original thesis, which remains unchanged. The author also incorporated current best practice concepts from national and international perspectives of health.

An Occupational Therapy Practice Model for the NICU

The following NICU practice model illustrates how *Achieving Growth and Development: An Expansion of Llorens' Developmental Theory of Occupational Therapy* guides practice in the NICU. As noted by Mitcham (2003), the logic of practice is defined by theory. This practice model is illustrated in Figure 13. Terminology is defined to clarify terms used in this model.

Description of Terms: These are concepts used to clarify the terms used in Figure 13.

1. Theory: This new theory that is depicted in Figure 13 is *Achieving Growth and Development: Premises and Concepts.* This theoretical model is based upon an expansion of Llorens' schematic model. Llorens provided premises and concepts related to the adaptation

FIGURE 13. Integrating Occupational Therapy Theory and Practice in the NICU. From Mitcham (2003, p. 81) (Adapted and reproduced with permission)

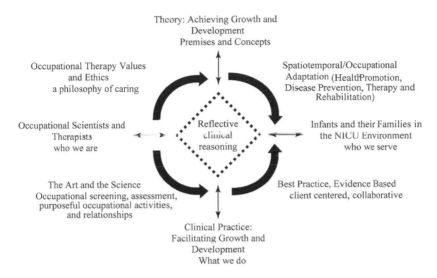

process in development throughout the lifespan. The expanded premises reflect additions to the Llorens' schematic model (Llorens, 1970).

2. Spatiotemporal and Occupational Adaptation: These terms (see Table 1) reflect the health promotion, disease prevention, therapy, and rehabilitation activities that provide a strategy for the "change process" needed to effect adaptive, healthful outcomes. This terminology is consistent with the AOTA's (2001) *Occupational Therapy in the Promotion of Health and the Prevention of Disease and Disability Statement.*

3. Infants and their Families in the NICU Environment: This term designates the population served by occupational therapy services in this work.

4. Best Practice, Evidence Based: This concept is defined as "client centered and collaborative" services, in that the occupational process (Figure 13) is based upon well-documented screening recommendations, evaluation techniques and assessment protocols, intervention techniques and measurable clinical outcomes

(including educational methods) as cited in the literature to provide the best possible results (AOTA, 2006).

5. Occupational Therapy Values and Ethics: This term refers to a
"philosophy of caring," which incorporates the focus of practice
and research; "do no harm," "informed consent." Additionally,
the philosophical values of the profession are included (AOTA,
2000).

6. Occupational Therapist and Scientist: This term identifies the
practitioner-scholar.

7. The Art and the Science: The process and logic of practice provides for occupational screening, assessment, purposeful occupational activities, and relationships in an *interactive process*
(Llorens, 1981b).

8. Clinical Practice: Achieving Growth and Development: Assessment of the infant's growth and development to build upon the
infant's and their family's strengths, starting from the point where
they are and following a developmental path through an occupational therapy process model (Figure 13).

9. Reflective Clinical Reasoning: This process of the practitioner-
scholar forms the basis for the practitioner's ability to assess
and to vary the levels of the treatment factor (intensity, timing,
duration, and frequency), and to successfully combine all aspects
of the model to translate theory into clinical practice for each
individual.

Professionalism in occupational therapy practice encompasses
critical thinking to analyze one's rationale for decisions, which are
based upon solid theoretical perspectives that can be articulated
(Parham, 1987). Theory is also essential to systematically evaluate
treatment methods, appraise intervention outcomes, disseminate
ideas for policy-making in health care, and validate existing theory
for further theory development efforts. The application of theory to
the process of occupational therapy practice is an expression of professional autonomy. Enhancing health through occupation "demon-
strates that the practitioner-scholar will give back to society a sound
body of knowledge, carefully evaluated services, and substantive
contributions to solving the health care problems of the nation"
(Parham, 1987, p. 555). Application of theory to practice requires
an occupational therapy process to achieve growth and development
of high-risk infants in the NICU that is evidenced based.

Occupational Therapy NICU Process Model in Health Promotion and Disease Prevention

Application of the developmental theory to the NICU can be viewed as a sequential process that guides practice. Its universality in depicting the need for occupational performance and participation from a developmental viewpoint in relevant contexts lends itself to the ICF's terminology (World Health Organization, 2001) to blend with the person occupation environment model. Personal and social outcomes of health conditions are based upon a person's participation in all areas of life. Categories of health are identified as primary, secondary, and tertiary prevention (World Health Organization, 1986) depending upon health care need. Key concepts from both the Healthy People's 2010 initiatives and from the World Health Organization recommend that practitioners screen high-risk infants for markers of cerebral palsy (Ferrari et al., 2002) or other neurodevelopmental sequelae (Majnemer, 2007; Majnemer, Rosenblatt, & Riley, 1994) as *preventable or manageable health conditions.*

Concepts from the ICF that pertain to the NICU, as conceptualized in *Achieving Growth and Development*, are (a) neuro behavioral organization of very low birth weight (VLBW) infants' body structures and functions (which encompass normal anatomical and occupationally physiological/psychological aspects of human beings) (Section 1 of Llorens), (b) participation in infant occupations of feeding, play, and social-caregiver interactions (Section 2 of Llorens), and (c) activity limitations in the NICU environment (Section 3 of Llorens).

An Occupational Therapy Process Model, derived from the *expanded* Developmental Theory of Occupational Therapy, explains why occupational therapists use activities (occupation) and relationships to predict outcomes of spatiotemporal and occupational adaptation in VLBW infants. As noted in the activity model of the ICF (Figure 11), the clinician prioritizes the infant's *Health Condition* in phases of wellness (Figure 14) to determine appropriate assessment and intervention strategy. Primary, secondary, and tertiary levels of prevention represent infant health care need.

Occupational therapy practice in the NICU, derived from the *Expanded Developmental Theory of Occupational Therapy,* as applied in a person, occupation, and environment process model, is as follows (see Figure 14).

Lynne F. La Corte

FIGURE 14. Occupational Therapy Practice in the NICU, Derived from the *Expanded Developmental Theory of Occupational Therapy*, as Applied in a Person, Occupation, and Environment Process Model

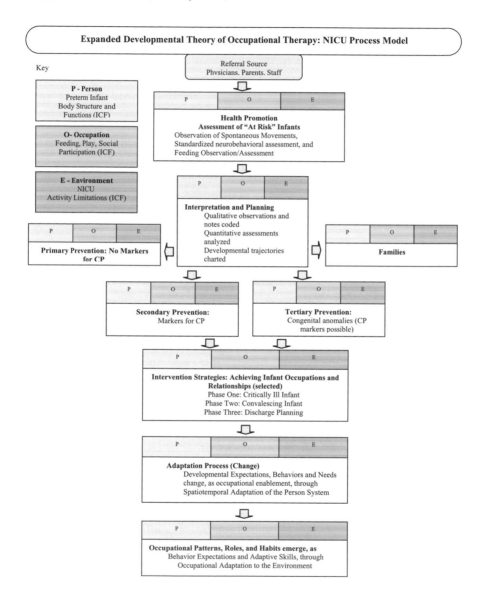

Application of the expanded *Developmental Theory of Occupational Therapy* predicts that the fundamental endowment of the individual and the stimulation of the experiences received within the environment of the family come together to interact in such a way as to promote positive early growth for both the individual family members and the family as a system. In the NICU context, the occupational therapist facilitates the spatiotemporal adaptation process through occupational activities, tasks, and relationships to culminate in an adaptive response becoming part of the system. Occupational adaptation acknowledges the physical, sociocultural, and psychodynamic influences (barriers and facilitators) of the NICU environment, in which newly learned responses and skills of infants and their families must be "occupationally meaningful" and, therefore, neurobehaviorally organizing.

In this highly technological environment, parents must often wait until specific visiting hours to see their infants and to sit in close proximity to their infant's crib or isolette. The infant is usually unable to respond to their parents while on a ventilator because of sedation, or the infant may be too fragile or ill to be held or have too many tubes or wires to be taken out of their beds. Therefore, the NICU environment disrupts child and family growth and development. The occupational therapist is an important link between infants and their families in the promotion of meaningful and purposeful relationships, activities, and environmental adaptation.

Practical Application of Theoretical Perspectives: Problem Identification and Solutions in Practice

Reed (1998) noted that all occupational therapy theories utilize four major concepts relevant to occupational endeavor, as person, environment, health, and occupation. *Achieving Growth and Development* brings a nonreductionistic (nonlinear) developmental perspective to bear upon these four concepts in an interrelated, interdependent, developmental theoretical framework (Hinojosa & Kramer, 1993). Although Llorens categorized various growth components individually to delineate how they enable occupational performance roles and participation in life, in actuality these components are dynamically interwoven developmental processes in which the whole is greater than the sum of its parts (Royeen, 2003;

Walker & Shortridge, 1993). As previously noted, the terminology used to describe an NICU occupational therapy program for children and their families from a developmental theory perspective of person, occupation, environment, and health should also reflect current terms and concepts from the World Health Organization's expanded health model (WHO, 2001).

Hinojosa and Kramer (1993) noted that theoretical frameworks provide "a methodological organization of theoretical and practical material in sequences needed for problem identification and solutions in practice" (Hinojosa & Kramer, 1993, p. 3). To apply perspectives from *Achieving Growth and Development* to an NICU program, the author provides a case illustration. This case describes care for an infant born at 22 weeks gestational age (GA) who is currently 37–38 weeks GA. This infant was diagnosed with early markers for a neurological impairment and has a nasogastric (NG) feeding tube. She is in the process of transitioning to oral feedings. The author includes current terminology used in the ICF in a person, occupation, and environment sequence, as related to infant, parent, and family health.

Achieving Growth and Development: The Infant

Person Factors: At 22 weeks GA, this pre-term infant struggles to cope with her environment. Her neurophysiological integrity is deficit for maintaining homeostasis. Sensory perception of tactile, vestibular, visual, auditory, olfactory, gustatory, proprioceptive, and kinesthetic sensations are poorly registered, interpreted, and integrated, possibly leading to a system deficit of the modulator aspects of occupation. This developmental disruption of an early birth with extremely low birth weight, along with neurological hemorrhage, lead to a system overload demonstrated by avoidance behaviors and increased agitation. Postural responses are often disorganized and inefficient in respect to the environment, affecting all body structures. Psychosocially, this infant's trust in the nurturance of sensory constancy has not been established, nor consistency in depth of sleep or ease of feeding. Positive responses from the infant to nurturing in the emotional regulation of affect are absent or diminished. Psychodynamically, the initiation of aggression associated with rooting for oral feeding is absent. In general, occupational performance enablers, which provide a basis for attachment and empathetic relationships, are negatively impacted in this infant. Change strategies will need to be directed toward these enablers of occupation, in addition to outcome occupational performance skills and relationships.

Occupations: From a sociocultural perspective, this infant is unable to occupationally engage in the oral erotic activity associated with feeding in response to bonding with the mother as the most important person, or to the immediate family group in play. During the NICU period, from critical to convalescent care, social language occupations for making small sounds, coos, vocalizations, and for visual pursuit and listening, are diminished, possibly due to time spent on the ventilator. Additionally, this infant's daily living occupation of feeding is poorly coordinated with the neurophysiological and sensory aspects of sucking, swallowing, and breathing. In general, the infant's participation in the family is negatively impacted by her occupational performance deficits. The parent involvement activities will need to focus upon change strategies in these areas.

Environment Factors: The environment presents a foreign physical, spatial, and temporal context for this infant, and it will need to be adapted to enhance her opportunities for occupational engagement. All of her developmental tasks in her environment are inhibited by her movement and sensory integrative limitations. Her responses to the environment for exploration and sensory perceptual experiences limit her play and social interactions. From an ego-adaptive viewpoint, this infant is unable to respond to mothering in her role of daughter, or to respond to the routines of daily living. The environment also inhibits the intellectual aspects involved in her motor skill integration. In general, the NICU and possibly, later, the home environment present barriers to her infant occupations and activities, which are significantly restricted. The parent participation activities will need to focus upon change strategies in these areas.

Achieving Growth and Development: The Parents

Person Factors: These parents continue to be challenged (from hospital to home environment) with a situation that is not easy for them to comprehend. Their difficulty coping with their infant's circumstances affects their neurophysiological functioning, creating stress. Their homeostasis is disrupted, possibly resulting in physical fatigue. Psychosocial aspects of occupational enablement to meet needs of commitment and partnership are impacted, and, psychodynamically, both parents find that their emotions are difficult to control. In general, these parents are in a state of shock due to a lack of strategies to efficiently cope with their child's needs, each other, and their own needs. They find they have shifted from comfort and enjoyment to survival-based needs.

Occupations: These parents' occupational roles for anticipated and expected participation in parenting were preempted by their child's early birth, and now by the child's neurological deficits. The sociocultural occupational performance skills usually involved with parenting are ineffectual with their child, and the parent's need for family group affiliation is unfulfilled. Parents confront unfamiliar social language, and the cognitive aspects of their child's care is unfamiliar. The occupational performance skills needed to understand and identify with their child's problems create difficulty for participation of infant caretaking routines. In general, these parents' occupational readiness for caretaking and understanding their neurologically involved infant to provide nurturance and mothering, comforting, playful interactions, and attachment behaviors are affected to varying degrees. All relationships are stressed, and coping mechanisms are diminished.

Environment Factors: From a temporal aspect, these parents' usual developmental tasks associated with work, leisure/play, and instrumental and basic maintenance daily occupations are imbalanced. Their lack of routines stress ego-adaptive behaviors needed to tolerate frustration, plan and execute, obtain, organize and use knowledge. From an intellectual viewpoint, parenting stresses present difficultly with a planned and systematic approach to problem-solving the parenting and spouse role. In general, the temporal environmental demands, which are occurring within their home environment, provide activity limitations for these parents in their ability to engage in balanced occupational roles, routines, and patterns associated with living.

Achieving Growth and Development: The Family

Application of an expanded developmental theory of occupational therapy predicts that the fundamental endowment of the individual and the stimulation of the experiences received within the environment of the family come together to interact in such a way as to promote positive early growth for both the individual family members and the family as a system. Therefore, a program for children and their families considers the occupational performance needs of family members and the family as an environment. The environment of family includes a family's aspirations, wants, goals, aims, priorities, and ambitions; in short, their culture. According to Llorens (1971), a family's culture provides the family with a means of coping with the external environment. The occupational therapist facilitates family growth and development by assisting the family in their ability to adjust to the demands of their culture and to achieve a sense of mastery in their occupational roles, routines, and habits (Llorens, 1971; AOTA, 2002).

Conclusion of Part 3

In conclusion, Part 3 of this book provided an application of new theorists to Llorens' model of *Facilitating Growth and Development*, in addition to application of revised psychodynamic components of activities and relationships and the application of the occupational physiology concept as the adaptive mechanism through which endogenous CPGs enable occupational performance components, activities, and roles. The organizational properties of CPGs provide for the enablement of spatiotemporal and occupational adaptation. Engineering, neurophysiologic, and animal behavior research support this proposition. Activity theory and growth models explain the value of purposeful activity and relationships in the achievement of growth and development, reinforcing the concept of the meaningfulness (themes of meaning) of everyday occupations. Last, current models and mandates in the quest for healthful outcomes were defined and applied in a practice-process model that addresses *Developmental Expectations, Behaviors, and Needs*, and *Behavior Expectation and Adaptive Skills* (Llorens, 1970) for infants and their families in the NICU. The author described a brief case illustration to explain a few of the major premises of the expanded theory. The final section of this issue focuses upon a data collection tool that utilizes a modified version of Llorens' data collection method for infants in the NICU. A similar modification of this same tool could provide a methodology to record assessment data for parents individually or for the family as an environment.

PART 4: THE DAEIS FOR RESEARCH AND
CLINICAL PRACTICE

In 1977, Llorens published the Occupational Therapy Developmental Analysis, Evaluation, and Intervention Schedule (DAEIS), as a sequential client record for the purpose of conducting research (Llorens, 1977b). And this record paradigmatically fits the developmental theory of occupational therapy that typifies congruent methods of measurement that could be, ideologically speaking, both explanatory and predictive within a given social context. In this manner, one might assert that science is based upon objective methodology that can be categorically defined for its meaning (data analysis) and theoretical comparability (interpretation), whereby conclusions could be drawn as symbolically significant (hypothetical interpretation) and new hypotheses suggested (speculation). According to Bandura (2003), "... humans have evolved an advanced cognitive capacity for observational learning that enables them to shape and structure their lives through the power of modeling" (p. 67). In the previous sections of this issue, the author presented models to explain continuums of function to dysfunction and to predict outcomes through the application of occupational activities and affective object relationships. The following data collection form, modified from Llorens' DAEIS (Llorens, 1977b), continues this paradigmatic fit in the Llorens tradition. Various frameworks and assessment tools that pertain to the theoretical constructs asserted in this theory expansion, such as Thelen's (1995) synthesis of motor development, could be utilized. The theoretical versatility of *The Developmental Theory of Occupational Therapy* provides an immense amount of flexibility to include multiple aspects of human development.

The NICU DAEIS form (used for research and adapted with permission from Llorens, 1977b) incorporates the following sections. In *Section 1* of the schedule, the individuals demographic information is recorded. In *Section II*, a history of postnatal complications scale is provided (modified from Littman and Parmelee, 1978). *Section III* provides for family demographics; *Section IV* lists the infant's occupational profile in terms of possible developmental disruptions in behaviors, expectations, and needs, and in behavior expectations and adaptive skills; these details serve to guide the choice of outcome measures. Evaluation techniques from procedures used are included in this section in addition to the evaluation data from the procedures used. Next is the Problem Identification of Section V, which notes the areas of occupational performance affected. This section includes a problems list for specific problems targeted for occupational therapy intervention. *Section VI* contains the therapy procedures indicated for maximum participation, as occupational therapy activities and relationships, and as physical and socio-cultural environmental modifications, along with the location of therapy. *Section VII* contains the narrative notes and the flow sheets to record intervention data, and *Section VIII* lists the discharge data as results of therapy noted from the various evaluation techniques and procedures and areas of occupational performance improved, maintained, or restored, and last, the infants disposition in respect to the date of discharge, final occupational plan, and follow-up pertaining to occupational therapy. The following record is specific to the NICU; however, one could easily modify it for other social contexts. The DAEIS could also be used for clinical practice.

Developmental Analysis, Evaluation, and Intervention Schedule for Infant and Family Occupations in the NICU (Research Form)

Section 1 Demographic Information: Birth History

Client's Name.	Date of Referral:	Date of First Treatment:	Case No:	Date of Birth:
Gestational Age at Birth:	Delivery:	Gender:	Age at Examination:	Referred by
Mother's Name:	Gravity:	Birth Order	Percentile.	SGA/AGA
Birth weight:	Birth length.	Apgar Score 1 min: (7-10 normal range)	Apgar Score 5 min: (7-10 normal range)	
Life Role:	Maternal drug History:			

Condition/Diagnosis:

Subjective:

Review of Systems

Neurological:

Cardiovascular:

Respiratory:

Social and communication:

Physical exam ongoing by physicians and NNPs:

Medications:

Reason for Referral: Subject in research study

Imaging

Head Ultrasound:

CAT SCAN/MRI Results:

Section II: History of Postnatal Complications: Score Each Condition as One Modified from Littman & Parmelee (1978)

Condition	Date/Comments	Date/Comments	Date/Comments	Total Score
Respiratory distress (CPAP, intubated)				
Ventilator/ECMO assistance (types, amount, and length of time in days)				
Infection				
Non-infectiousillness (anomaly, hemorrhage >3, acute or cystic PVL, other				
Metabolic abnormality				
Convulsion				
Hyperbilirubinemia or exchange transfusion				
Temperature disturbance				
First feeding within 48 hours of birth (score as 1 if no)				
Surgery				

Section III: Family Demographics

Condition/Family Member	Characteristic: Circle Choice	Additional Information
Mother's education	10–12 yr	
	High School/GED	
	Some college	
	Bachelor's degree	
	Graduate degree	
Mother's age		
Mother's work status	Full–time	
	Part-time	
	No work	
Mother's ethnicity	White	
	Black	
	Hispanic	
	Asian	
	Other	
Mother born in the United States	Yes	
	No	
Father's education (name is Hugo)	10–12 yr	
	High School/GED	
	Some college	
	Bachelor's degree	
	Graduate degree	
Father's age		
Father's work status	Full-time	
	Part-time	
	No work	
Father's ethnicity	White	
	Black	
	Hispanic	
	Asian	
	Other	
Father born in the United States	Yes	
	No	
Mother's Marital Status	Single	
	Married	
Family Income	<$10,000	
	$10,000–$25,000	
	$25,000–$50,000	
	$50,000–$75,000	
	$75,000–$100,000	
	>$100,000	
Insurance	HMO/private	
	Medicaid/government	
	Self/None	
Mother's prenatal visits	None	
	1–3	
	3–5	
	>5	

Section IV: Growth and Development Disruptions of Occupational Engagement (participation) in daily activities relative to age, gender, life role, and condition in (a) body structures and functions for occupational enablement (developmental needs, behaviors, and expectations) and in (b) contextual environmental adaptation (socio-cultural and physical behavior expectations and adaptive skills).

Occupational Profile

(Possible developmental disruptions relative to age, gender, life role, and condition)

Developmental Behaviors, Expectations, and Needs

Neurophysiological: For example, risk factors along with metabolic, congential, genetic, and organic damage to efficient and adaptive processing/modulation that compromise all areas of development.

Physical: For example, maintaining open airways, organ support in general, positioning, and structural deficits.

Psychosocial: For example, the effect of multiple caregivers due to the NICU environment, which affects attachment. Often procedures are provided without any warning to the infant.

Psychodynamic: For example, psychosexual state of oral feeding is compromised, and attachment to maternal and circadian rhythms are compromised, along with the neuro-physiological aspects of affective growth and development.

Sociocultural: For example, NICU sounds and languages provide a variety of cultural orientation. Parents visiting hours are often limited, which often means limited parenting.

Social Language: For example, containment with rocking, along with sucking on the pacifier, are used to decrease stress, also sugar as "sweeties" for painful procedures.

Activities of Daily Living: For example, caregiver interactions (holding and rocking) and "cares" are frequently performed by nursing (changing diaper, feeding is at times with a bottle or a nasogastric tube and/TPN [intravenous], and taking temperatures), with or without parental involvement for cares.

Behavior Expectations and Adaptive Skills

Ego-Adaptive Skills: For example, personality development and coping mechanisms are affected by the constraints of the environment, the lack of an integrated system for breathing, movement and feeding, and various environmental restrictions for sensorimotor exploration, attachment, and bonding.

Developmental Tasks: For example, occupational roles and engagement in areas of occupation are delayed due to the critical care needs (play, feeding, learning, attachment, care-giving interactions).

Human Ecology: For example, establishing mutually rewarding relationships.

Discovery Learning: For example, motor learning of action sequences.

Intellectual: For example, the integration of motor skills within environmental context of home is absent.

Evaluation Techniques and Procedures Indicated (List):

Behaviour Observations   Interview   Review of History   Testing

Evaluation Data from Procedures Used (Findings):

Data(s) of Evaluation –

Behavior Observations –

Interview Data –

History –

Tests/Evaluations Used and Findings –

Section V – Problem Identification: Areas of Occupational Performance Affected (List):

Consider capabilities and engagement (participation) in activities and relationships

1. Child-Adult Self-Care: Neonatal – feeding, caregiver interactions and procurement for care-giving and regulatory needs.
2. Child-Adult Education (learning)/Work: Neonatal – state control, orientation to animate and inanimate objects, self regulatory abilities.
3. Play/Leisure: Neonatal – procuring, visual and auditory exploration, crying -playing with sounds for communicative purposes, occupational routines, habits and patterns – occupational behaviors.
4. Rest: Neonatal – sleep-rest cycles, circadian rhythm

Problems List *(Specific problems indicated for occupational therapy intervention)*:

Section VI – Occupational Therapy Activity and Relationship Plan (Specific objectives keyed to problems list):

1. Specific Objectives Keyed to Problem List:
2. Therapy Procedures indicated for maximum participation (Activities and Relationships indicated):
3. Physical and Socio-Cultural Environmental Modifications: Environmental limitations and barriers, needed adaptations, and socio-cultural contextual factors:

4. Location of Therapy: (Where and when):

Section VII – Progress Notes

See attached Flow Sheets and Narrative Notes

Section VIII I: Final Results

Results of Therapy (List indicated procedures)

Behavior Observations

Interview

Review of History

Testing

Reevaluation Data from Procedures Used (Finding dates):

Areas of Occupational Performance Improved, Maintained or Restored (List):

1. Child-Adult Self-Care: Neonatal – feeding, caregiver interactions and procurement for care-giving and regulatory needs.
2. Child-Adult Education (learning)/Work: Neonatal – state control, orientation to animate and inanimate objects, self regulatory abilities.
3. Play/Leisure: Neonatal – procuring, visual and auditory exploration, crying -playing with sounds for communicative purposes,

occupational routines, habits and patterns – occupational behaviors.
4. Rest: Neonatal – sleep-rest cycles, circadian rhythm.

Disposition:

• Date of Discharge –

• Occupational Plan -

• Follow-up

Signature_____ Date_____

Progress and Narrative Notes (keyed to problem list in *Section V* and dated):

S – subjective...

O – objective...

A – assessment...

P – plan...

Flow Sheets (keyed to problem list in *Section V* and dated, one sheet may be used for each plan):

| PLANS: | | | | | | | | | | | | | | | COMMENTS: |

Therapy Procedures	1	2	3	4	4	5	6	7	8	9	10	11	12	13	14	Heart Rate, Respiration and FiO_2

Next, the author provides a case illustration of how the DAEIS could be utilized for clinical practice.

Developmental Analysis, Evaluation, and Intervention Schedule for Infant and Family Occupations in the NICU
(Research Form, version 1.3)

Section 1—Demographic Information: Birth History

Condition/Diagnosis (description from reference source): Subjective 2/12/08: Former 22-week-old female infant with CLD (chronic lung disease). History of 2 bowel perforations with creation of mucus fistula and ostomy. Infant with functional short bowel secondary

Client's Name: Baby A   **Date of Referral:** 2/1/08   **Date of First Treatment:** 2/6/08

Case No: A   **Date of Birth:** 10/10/2007   **Gestational Age at Birth:** 22 weeks

Delivery: Vaginal Birth

Gender: F   **Mother's Name:** Mariana   **Gravity:** 1   **Birth Order:** 1   **Age at**

Examination: 38 weeks   **Birth weight:** 600 grams   **Birth length:** 30 cm. **Apgar Score:**

1 min (7-10 normal range) 7   **Apgar Score:** 5 min (7-10 normal range) 7

Percentile:AGA = 10th percentile

to high ostomy with enteral feeding intolerance. Stable work of breathing on NC (nasal canula). Occasional A/B/Ds (apnea/brady-bradycardia/desaturations). Takedown surgery (Reanastomosis [reestablishing bowel continuity]) planned per Dr. D approximately 2/20/08. Infant currently receives TPN (total parenteral nutrition [intravenous feeding]) and small volume feedings for nutritional support.

Problem: On Prevacid for clinical signs of GER (gastroesophageal reflux).

Cardiovascular access: Infant with long-term IV access needs for nutritional support, currently located in SVC (superior vena cava).

Problem: Respiratory

- Respiratory Distress: History of surfactant modified RDS, now with mild, slowly improving CLD. Infant currently (2/12) on NC at 1 LPM (liter per minute); FiO_2 (fractionated oxygen saturation) = 0.23 0, low and stable. Flow weaning gradually, titrate FiO_2 to maintain SaO_2 (saturation level) 88–95%.
- Infant with apnea most likely due to prematurity. Caffeine therapy continues despite approx. 38 weeks adjusted gestation as she had increased apnea when caffeine was stopped. Last attempt to discontinue caffeine took place 1/14/08. No spells requiring medical intervention the last couple of weeks.

Problem: Pain and sedation: ongoing

Problem: Bowel perforation: Infant with small bowel perforation; repaired in the OR on 10/19. Ileostomy created. 11/17/07 had secondary bowel perforation below initial ostomy. 6-cm ileum resected.

Social and Communication: Social Worker in touch with parents, who mainly speak Spanish. Extended family support noted.

Problem: Mild anemia/hyperbilirubinemia.

Head Ultrasound: No evidence of IVH on serial HUS. MRI done 11/29/07. The lissencephalic appearance of the brain is in keeping with the age adjustment at 27 weeks. Small focal left lateral cerebellar hemosiderin deposit consistent with remote probable germinal matrix bleed. Developmental hypoplasia of the right transverse and right sigmoid venous sinus. OFC (occipital facial circumference) growth 10% percentile, consistent with infant's overall growth.

Physical Exam: Ongoing by physicians and neonatal nurse practitioners.

Medications: See above, changed as needed by physician.

Reason for Referral: Developmental evaluation to include oral motor coordination (suck, swallow, breath) for feeding.

Referred by: Dr. N

Life Role: Daughter

Imaging Results: See HUS (head ultrasound) and MRI above

Maternal Drug History: None

Surgery: "Takedown" planned for 2/20. Infant will be NPO (nothing by mouth) and intubated. Oral feeding will hopefully be reestablished per physician's order sometime soon after the surgery.

Section II: History of Postnatal Complications: Score Each Condition as One Modified from Littman & Parmelee (1978)

Condition	Date/Comments	Date/Comments	Date/Comments	Total Score
Respiratory distress (CPAP, intubated)	10/10 /07			
Ventilator/ECMO assistance (types, amount, and length of time in days)	10/10/07	2/20 for surgery		
Infection	12/2/07			
Non-infectious illness (anomaly, hemorrhage >3, acute or cystic PVL, other	11/29 germinal matrix hemorrhage noted on MRI			
Metabolic abnormality				
Convulsion	10/25 seizure activity			
Hyperbilirubinemia or exchange transfusion				
Temperature disturbance	X			
First feeding within 48 hours of birth (score as 1 if no)	X			
Surgery	11/2 bowel resection due to perforation	2/20 reanastomosis		
Comments:				

Section III: Family Demographics

Condition/Family Member	Characteristic: Circle Choice	Additional Information
Mother's education	10–12 years	Mother is from Mexico
	High School/GED	Some high school
	Some college	
	Bachelor's degree	
	Graduate degree	
Mother's age	17	
Mother's work status	Full-time	No
	Part-time	
	No work	
Mother's ethnicity	White	
	Black	
	Hispanic	X Mother speaks mainly Spanish and a little English
	Asian	
	Other	
Mother born in the United States	Yes	
	No	X
Father's education	10–12 years	Father is from Mexico
	High School/GED	Some high school
	Some college	
	Bachelor's degree	
	Graduate degree	
Father's age	20	
Father's work status	Full-time	
	Part-time	
	No work	
Father's ethnicity	White	
	Black	
	Hispanic	X Father speaks mainly Spanish
	Asian	
	Other	
Father born in the United States	Yes	
	No	X
Mother's Marital Status	Single	
	Married	X
Family Income	<$10,000	
	$10,000–$25,000	X
	$25,000–$50,000	
	$50,000–$75,000	
	$75,000–$100,000	
	>$100,000	
Insurance	HMO/private	
	Medicaid/government	X
	Self/none	
Mother's prenatal visits	None	
	1–3	X
	3–5	
	>5	

Section IV: Growth and Development Disruptions of Occupational Engagement (participation) in daily activities relative to age, gender, life role, and condition in (a) body structures and functions for occupational enablement (developmental needs, behaviors, and expectations) and in (b) contextual environmental adaptation (socio-cultural and physical behavior expectations and adaptive skills).

Occupational Profile

(Possible developmental disruptions relative to age, gender, life role, and condition)

Developmental Behaviors, Expectations and Needs

Neurophysiological: The gestational age and germinal matrix hemorrhage of baby A present risk factors for all areas of development.

Physical: Maintaining open airways, periodic breathing; apnea and bradycardia are present, organ support is necessary.

Psychosocial: Infant has multiple caregivers due to the NICU environment which could affect attachment. Procedures may be provided without any warning to the infant.

Psychodynamic: Psychosexual state of oral feeding is compromised, attachment to maternal figure and circadian rhythms are compromised, along with the neuro-physiological aspects of growth and development.

Sociocultural: NICU sounds provide a variety of cultural orientations. Parents visit on weekends; have difficulty with transportation and need to have their parents bring them to visit their daughter. Limited parenting at this time.

Social Language: Reciprocity and social learning opportunities are absent.

Activities of Daily Living: Caregiver interactions (holding and rocking); "cares" (changing diaper, feeding is enteral and TPN, taking temperature, measurements of girth) are performed mainly by nursing personnel, with occupational therapy consultation for parental involvement when possible (parent availability). Oral feeding has been established on a minimal basis.

Behavior Expectations and Adaptive Skills

Ego-Adaptive Skills: Personality development and coping mechanisms could be affected by the constraints of the environment, the lack of an integrated system for breathing, movement, and feeding, and various environmental restrictions for sensorimotor exploration, attachment, and bonding.

Developmental Tasks: Occupational roles and engagement in areas of occupation (play, feeding, learning, attachment, care-giving interactions) could be delayed due to the critical care needs of this infant.

Human Ecology: The establishment of mutually rewarding relationships is delayed.

Discovery Learning: The motor learning of action sequences could be somewhat delayed.

Intellectual: The integration of motor skills within environmental context of home is absent.

Evaluation Techniques and Procedures Indicated (List):

Behaviour Observations X   Interview X   Review of History X   Testing X

Evaluation Data from Procedures Used (Findings):

Data(s) of Evaluation—2/1/08

Behavior Observations—

- Infant "Cares": Behavioral observations were made during "cares"; the infant becomes quite agitated; often her oxygen level needs increased.
- Oral motor coordination: Swallow does not appear automatic when therapist touches the peri-oral or the intra-oral musculature. Additionally, infant tends to hold her breath when touched in these areas.
- Bottle Feeding: This infant has received small feeds, and her feeding pattern reveals chomping, biting movements, where breathing is not well coordinated with sucking and especially swallowing.

Frequent desaturations during feeding and need for increased FiO$_2$.
- Spontaneous Movements: This infant's initial qualitative trajectory revealed camped synchronized movements (Prechtl's Qualitative Method).

Interview Data: The parents speak Spanish fluently. They are living with their relatives, and the father works in a restaurant. An interpreter is needed.

History: This infant has been on caffeine and various antibiotics (see above history for additional information).

Tests Used and Findings: Behavioral trajectory from Prechtl's Qualitative Method (as noted above under spontaneous movements) indicated camped synchronized movements (where there is an "all or none" type of response in the extremities and trunk). Other standardized assessments: The Brazelton Neonatal Behavioral Assessment Scale, 3rd Edition (BNBAS, completed as possible). Motor processes were deficit; Interactive processes were deficit; Organizational—physiological response to stress was deficit, and Organizational—state control was deficit.

Section V: Problem Identification: Areas of Occupational Performance Affected (List)

Consider capabilities and engagement (participation) in activities and relationships.

1. Child-Adult Self-Care: Neonatal—feeding, caregiver interactions, and procurement for care-giving and regulatory needs.
2. Child-Adult Education (Learning)/Work: Neonatal—state control, orientation to animate and inanimate objects, self-regulatory abilities.
3. Play/Leisure: Neonatal—procuring, visual and auditory exploration, crying—playing with sounds for communicative purposes, occupational routines, habits and patterns, occupational behaviors.
4. Rest: Neonatal—sleep-rest cycles, circadian rhythm. Pain medication for sleep.

Problems List (Specific problems indicated for occupational therapy intervention):

All areas of occupational performance (capabilities) and engagement (participation) are compromised; in particular

1. Interpreter needed during all interactions with parents, including parent collaboration and participation.
2. Feeding (caregiver interactions): The feeding pattern is poorly coordinated, and there is pocketing of the liquid bolus, perhaps to allow for breathing, which does not appear coordinated with sucking and swallowing. Also, tremulous 1/2 sucks (sips) include a tongue thrust. Coordination appears poor for tongue, lip, and jaw movements that are needed for an efficient suck, swallow, and breathe synergy. Oral hypersensitivity is also noted. There appears to be a rigid quality to the infant's muscle tone on her developmental trajectory that probably affects her oral motor coordination.
3. Learning: (a) State control, attention: difficulty maintaining states of alertness with postural control, without agitation, which is probably related to (b) self-regulation: difficulty with neural modulation of states, including emotionality. Postural integration appears poorly coordinated in regard to spontaneous and elicited movements, and therefore not well integrated with interactive or attentional abilities.
4. Play: Limited sensory exploration. Infant is contained in a bendy bumper, unavailable for visual and auditory exploration, tactile exploration, movement exploration, or the establishment of relationships. The IV lines, tubes, and monitoring equipment present an environmental limitation.
5. Rest/relaxation: NICU routines are not the same as infants receive in utero and later on at home. Rest is sometimes interrupted with painful procedures, which make restful sleep difficult.

Section VI: Occupational Therapy Activity and Relationship Plan
Specific Objectives Keyed to Problem List

1. Improve oral motor coordination and feeding abilities.
2. Enhance movement organization and coupling of posture with state control and attention.
3. Provide positioning for play.

4. Enhance parental opportunities for collaboration and participation.

Therapy Procedures Indicated for Maximum Participation: Activities and Relationships Indicated

1. Oral motor and feeding activities for oral discrimination, coordination, and for an efficient suck, swallow, and breathe pattern during bottle feeding.

   a. Parent training in these activities prior to and during feeding.

2. Activities for movement organization paired with state control and attention
   a. Containment to calm the infant and decrease stress

   b. Non-nutritive sucking, hands to mouth
   c. Parent participation and interaction with the infant during "cares"

   d. Infant massage activities with parent and infant
   e. Postural organization activities on the parent's lap or at the shoulder, paired with rocking and containment, which appear to calm the infant.
   f. Parent and infant interaction as possible for visual and auditory orientation and for snuggling.

Physical and Socio-Cultural Environmental Modifications: Environmental Limitations and Barriers, Needed Adaptations, and Socio-Cultural Contextual Factors

1. In addition to "nesting" and "containment" (swaddling), use of a baby chair (on a wire frame, which is similar to a hammock and sometimes called a baby "bounce" chair), that gently swings or bounces, and monitored prone positioning.
2. Mobiles, music, mirrors.
3. Gel pack pillow used as needed as a positional device.

Location of Therapy: In the NICU

Section VII: Progress Notes

Flow Sheets and Progress Notes were kept for the record.

Section VIII: Final Results:

Results of Therapy

Behavior Observations:

- Infant "Cares": Behavioral observations were made during "cares"; the infant is on room air and tolerates handling without agitation. Eye contact, smiles, auditory localization are all excellent.
- Oral motor coordination: The infant localized well to the selected sensory input with her tongue (when the therapist applied selected sensory input, per the intervention plan, to both the peri-oral and the intra-oral musculature). Swallowing has become automatic during the oral motor coordination facilitation activities and appears well coordinated with breathing and sucking.
- Bottle Feeding: This infant is up to full feeds and the NG tube is out. She exhibits good coordination during feeding, with a 1:1 suck/swallow pattern. Breathing appears well integrated with sucking and swallowing, and the infant self-paces well during the feeding. No FiO_2 desaturations have been noted during feeding for some time.
- Spontaneous Movements: This infant's qualitative developmental trajectory observation revealed a poor repertoire of movements, with good hand to mouth and "batting" movements noted.

Interview Data: During the exit interview, the parents concluded that they felt competent to care for, interact with, calm, and feed their infant. They also noted that they felt the occupational therapy intervention had improved the infant's feeding, general oral motor coordination, along with postural coordination paired with attention and interactions with the caregiver. Parents noted that infant exhibited restful sleep after the infant massage. When asked how the intervention could be improved, the parents said that they could not think of any additional activities or procedures to add to the intervention.

History: This infant has received her second surgery, namely a reanastomosis, and progressed to full oral feeding.

Tests Used and Findings: Developmental motor behavior trajectory from Prechtl's Qualitative Method (as noted above under spontaneous movements) indicated an improvement from cramped synchronized to a poor repertoire of movements with the emergence of isolated and rotational movements in the extremities.

Other standardized assessments included the Brazelton Neonatal Behavioral Assessment Scale, 3rd Edition (BNBAS). Motor processes, interactive processes, organizational—physiological response to stress, and organizational—state control were all within normal limits.

Reevaluation Data from Procedures Used:

Areas of Occupational Performance Improved (In this illustration, all areas improved. In particular, see specific results of the intervention outcome measures, noted above):

* Child-Adult Self-Care: Neonatal—feeding, caregiver interactions, and procurement for care-giving and regulatory needs.
* Child-Adult Education (Learning)/Work: Neonatal—state control, orientation to animate and inanimate objects, self-regulatory abilities.
* Play/Leisure: Neonatal—procuring, visual and auditory exploration, crying—playing with sounds for communicative purposes, occupational routines, habits and patterns, occupational behaviors.
* Rest: Neonatal—sleep-rest cycles, circadian rhythm.

Disposition

* Date of Discharge: 3/24/08
* Occupational Plan: Parents were provided with written instructions, with demonstration by the therapist, and a return demonstration provided by the parents of home program activities per the above activities.
* Follow-up related to OT: Infant will be seen in an early intervention home-based program to include occupational therapy.

Signature _____
Date _____

Conclusion of Part 4

In the final section of this issue, the author presented a modified version of Llorens' record-keeping form that brings together the pivotal aspects of the expanded theory of achieving growth and development. This kind of a check-back system reinforces the theory to research/practice paradigm: the evaluation tool must reflect the theoretical premises and constructs of its theoretical basis. The flexibility of the DAEIS lies in its links with the theoretical constructs of the *expanded developmental theory of occupational therapy*, without dictating a specific type of interview form or technique, behavior observation, historical review, or type of assessment/testing tool. Additionally, one could insert additional theorists/concepts (neurophysiologic, for example) into the expanded model (as was done here), with an explanation of its fit with the model under each of the POE areas as needed. In other words, this expanded model (and albeit its predecessor) serve as an umbrella for other theories, frameworks, or practice models.

The congruence of the DAEIS with its corresponding theory lies in the clustering of components for analysis, interpretation, and conclusions as reflected in the theory. In other words, have growth and development been achieved in the infant/family developmental needs, behaviors, and expectations as *occupational enablement* for *spatiotemporal adaptation*; and have growth and development been achieved in the infant/family behavior expectations and adaptive skills as *contextual occupational adaptation*?

Conclusion of Review, Update, and Expansion of Llorens

In closing, the author has evaluated, analyzed, and synthesized the theoretical and conceptual framework of Llorens. More recent developmental models, based upon theorists such as Bandura, Bronfenbrenner, Bruner, Peck and Havighurst, Freud, Moore, and von Holst were evaluated, analyzed, and applied to the Llorens model. For example, Bandura's research supports performance-based learning and the positive role of occupational enablement and environmental entrainment through social cognition. Bruner's focus upon discovery learning underscores the developmental pathway to one's *occupational self* through constructivism. Peck and Havighurst equilibrated Freud's psychosexual personality stages to moral character development. Additionally, research has shed new light on psychoanalytic theory and process. Moore's expansion of McLean's triune constructs illustrate the evolutionary aspects involved in the integrated nature of learning. And, newer constructs in the realm of CPG research and concepts provides an in-depth perspective on the role of occupational physiology in the adaptation process.

The NICU as a practice area for occupational therapists came about in the late 1960s. The initial focus was upon specific kinds of disability or problems with positioning. Occupational therapists have consistently addressed the infant occupation of feeding and positioning in the NICU as aspects of infant/caregiver self-care (Hunter, 2005). In the 1980s, occupational therapy's practice addressed more specific needs for neuromotor organization for those infants considered "at risk" for neurodevelopmental impairment and feeding deficits (Case-Smith, 1988). With the advent of developmental care, occupational therapists realized that, in addition to neurodevelopmental treatment techniques to enhance neuromotor organization for feeding, the use of swaddling and specific neurodevelopmental handling techniques to promote movement organization and to contain infants are also neurologically organizing and seem to promote rest, state control, transitions between states, and build relationships through enhanced attentional capacity for the infant's social cognition. The facilitation of neuromotor organization as discussed above for feeding and movement is utilized to enhance sensorimotor processing for intra/ interhemispheric integration as a reflection of the brain's capacity for healing through neuroplasticity. To achieve adaptive infant and family growth and development, the author applied health promotion and disease prevention concepts to theoretical practice and process models for application of occupational therapy practice in the NICU. In so doing, she also recognized the relevance of WHO's ICF for neonates. Additionally, the author recognized the psychosocial dimension of participation in activity, as delineated in the ICF by WHO, for the family, infant, and therapist relationship.

Purposeful activities in the NICU such as feeding, care giving, and communication through holding, looking, caressing, and grooming provide a basis for dyadic reciprocity of appropriate object relationships and affective responses.

Last, the author presented a modified version of the DAEIS as a methodological system to record, analyze, interpret, and conclude the effects of an occupational therapy intervention. The DAEIS fulfills the paradigmatic requirements of a true theory.

ACKNOWLEDGMENT

The author would like to thank George Kemenes, Ph.D., Professor of Neuroscience, Sussex Centre for Neuroscience, School of Life Sciences, University of Sussex, Falmer, Brighton, U.K.; and Pete Redgrave, Ph.D., Professor of Neuroscience, Neuroscience Research Unit, Dept. of Psychology, University of Sheffield, Sheffield, U.K, for their professional and editorial guidance.

REFERENCES

Akay, M., Lipping, T., Moodie, K., & Hoopes, P. J. (2002). Effects of hypoxia on the complexity of respiratory patterns. *Early Human Development, 70,* 55–71.

Als, H. (1989). Self-regulation and motor development in preterm infants. In J. Lockman (Ed.), *Action in social context* (pp. 81–83). New York: Plenum Press.

American Occupational Therapy Association. (1979). The philosophical base of occupational therapy. *American Journal of Occupational Therapy, 33,* 785.

American Occupational Therapy Association. (2000). Occupational therapy code of ethics. *American Journal of Occupational Therapy, 54,* 614–616.

American Occupational Therapy Association. (2001). Occupational therapy in the promotion of health and the prevention of disease and disability statement. (2001 addendum to the reference manual of the official documents of the American Occupational Therapy Association, Inc.). Bethesda, MD: American Occupational Therapy Association.

American Occupational Therapy Association. (2006). Specialized knowledge and skills in the neonatal intensive care unit. *American Journal of Occupational Therapy, 60*(6), 659–668.

American Occupational Therapy Association. (2007). Specialized knowledge and skills in feeding, eating, and swallowing for occupational therapy practice. *American Journal Occupational Therapy, 61*(6), 686–700.

Arshavsky, Y. I. (2003). Cellular and network properties in the functioning of the nervous system: From central pattern generators to cognition. *Brain Research— Brain Research Reviews, 41,* 229–267.

Arshavsky, Y., Deliagina, T. G., & Orlovsky, G. N. (1997). Pattern generation. *Current Opinion in Neurobiology, 7*, 781–789.

Ayres, A. J. (1974). Occupational therapy for motor disorders resulting from impairment to the central nervous system. In A. Henderson, L. Llorens, E. Gilfoyle, C. Myers & S. Prevel (Eds.), *The development of sensory integrative theory and practice*. Dubuque, Iowa: Kendall/Hunt (Reprinted from: Occupational therapy for motor disorders resulting from impairment to the central nervous system. Rehabilitation Literature, 1960, 21, 302–310)..

Ayres, A. J. (1972). Sensory integration and learning disorders. Los Angeles: Western Psychological Services.

Ayres, A. J. (1974). Occupational therapy for motor disorders resulting from impairment to the central nervous system. In A. Henderson, L. Llorens, E. Gilfoyle, C. Myers, & S. Prevel (Eds.), *The development of sensory integrative theory and practice*. Dubuque, IA: Kendall/Hunt (Reprinted from: Occupational therapy for motor disorders resulting from impairment to the central nervous system. *Rehabilitation Literature, 1960, 21*, 302–310).

Bandura, A. (1977a). *Social learning theory*. New Jersey: Prentice-Hall.

Bandura, A. (1977b). Self-efficacy: Toward a unifying theory of behavior change. *Psychological Review, 84*, 191–215.

Bandura, A. (1994). Self-efficacy. Retrieved December 13, 2004, from http://www.emory.edu/EDUCATION/mfp/BanEncy.html (Reprinted in: *Encyclopedia of Mental Health*, Vol. 4, pp. 71–78, H. Friedman (Ed.), 1998, San Diego, CA: Academic Press).

Bandura, A. (2003). On the psychosocial impact and mechanisms of spiritual modeling. *International Journal for the Psychology of Religion, 13*, 167–174.

Bandura, A. (2004). Health promotion by social cognitive means. *Health Education & Behavior: The Official Publication of the Society for Public Health Education, 31*, 143–164.

Bandura, A., Caprara, G. V., Barbaranelli, C., Gerbino, M., & Pastorelli, C. (2003). Role of affective self-regulatory efficacy in diverse spheres of psychosocial functioning. *Child Development, 74*(3), 769–783.

Bax, M., Goldstein, M., Rosenbaum, P., Leviton, A., Paneth, N., Dan, B., et al. (2005). Proposed definition and classification of cerebral palsy, April 2005. *Developmental Medicine and Child Neurology, 47*(8), 571.

Baum, C., & Law, M. (1997). Occupational therapy practice: Focusing on occupational performance. *The American Journal of Occupational Therapy, 51*, 287–288.

Bazyk, S. (1990). Factors associated with the transition to oral feeding in infants fed by nasogastric tubes. *American Journal of Occupational Therapy, 44*, 1070–1078.

Bem, T., Cabelguen, J.-M., Ekeberg, O., & Grillner, S. (2003). From swimming to walking: A single basic network for two different behaviors. *Biological Cybernetics, 88*(2), 79–90.

Benjamin, P. R., Staras, K., & Kemenes, G. (2000). A systems approach to the cellular analysis of associative learning in the pond snail lymnaea. *Learning and Memory, 7*, 124–131.

Bennett, F. C., & Scott, D. (1997). Long-term perspective on premature infant outcome and contemporary intervention issues. *Seminars in Perinatology, 21*, 190–201.

Bernstein, N. (1967). *Co-ordination and regulation of movements.* New York: Pergamon Press.

Bhutta, A. T., Cleves, M. A., Casey, P., Cradock, M. M., & Annand, J. K. S. (2002). Cognitive and behavioral outcomes of school-aged children who were born preterm: A meta-analysis. *The Journal of the American Medical Association, 288*, 728–737.

Bjorklund, D. F. (1997). The role of immaturity in human development. *Psychological Bulletin, 122*, 153–169.

Bobath, B. (1954). A study of abnormal postural reflex activity in patients with lesions of the central nervous system, I. *Physiotherapy, 40*, 259–300.

Bockting, W. O., & Coleman, E. (2003). *Masturbation as a means of achieving sexual health.* NY: Haworth Press.

Breger, L. (2000). *Freud: Darkness in the midst of vision.* New York: John Wiley & Sons.

Bronfenbrenner, U. (1975). *Influences on human development.* Hinsdale, IL: Dryden Press.

Brofenenbrenner, U. (1977). Toward an experimental ecology of human development. *American Psychologist, 32*(7), 513–531.

Brofenenbrenner, U. (1979). *The ecology of human development: Experiments by nature and design.* Cambridge, MA: Harvard University Press.

Bronfenbrenner, U. (2000). Ecological systems theory. In A. E. Kazdin. (Ed.), *Encyclopedia of psychology*, (Vol. 3, pp. 129–133). Washington, DC: American Psychological Association Oxford University Press.

Bronfenbrenner, U., & Ceci, S. J. (1994). Nature-nuture reconceptualized in developmental perspective: A bioecological model. *Psychological Review, 101*, 568–586.

Bronfenbrenner, U., & Morris, P. A. (1998). The ecology of developmental processes. In R. M. Lerner. (Ed.), *Handbook of child psychology: Theoretical models of human development,* (5th ed., Vol. 1, pp. 993–1028). New York: Wiley.

Brooks, V. (1986). *The neural basis of motor control.* London: Oxford Press.

Bruner, J. S. (1965). The growth of mind. *American Psychologist, 20*, 1007–1017.

Bruner, J. S. (1966). *Toward a theory of instruction.* New York: Norton.

Bruner, J. S. (1973). Organization of early skilled action. *Child Development, 44*, 1–11.

Bruner, J. S. (1975). The ontogenesis of speech acts. *Journal of Child Language, 2*, 1–19.

Bruner, J. S. (1976). Nature and uses of immaturity. In J. Brunner, A. Jolly, & K. Silava. (Eds.), *Play: Its role in development and evolution*, (pp. 29–67). New York: Basic Books.

Bruner, J. S. (1999). Infancy and culture: A story. In M. H. S. Chaiklin et al.. (Eds.), *Activity theory and social practice*, (pp. 225–234). Aarhus, Denmark: Aarhus University Press.

Bundy, A. C., Lane, S. J., & Murray, E. A. (2002). *Sensory integration theory and practice*. Philadephia: F. A. Davis.

Care Connection for Children. (2007). Retrieved March 13, 2008, from http://www.careconnections.vcu.edu/2010.html

Caretto, V., Topolski, K., Linkous, C., Lowman, K., & Murphy, S. (2000). Current parent education on feeding in the neonatal intensive care unit: The role of the occupational therapist. *American Journal Occupational Therapy, 54*, 59–64.

Case-Smith, J. (Ed.). (2005). *Occupational therapy for children* (5 ed.). St Louis: Mosby.

Cohen, A. (1992). The role of heterarchical control in the evolution of central pattern generators. *Brain Behavior Evolution, 40*, 112–124.

Cohen, H. (1999). *Neuroscience for rehabilitation* (2nd ed.). Philadelphia: Lippincott, Williams & Wilkins.

Coles, R. (Ed.). (2000). *The Erik Erikson reader*. New York: WWW Norton & Company.

Commissiong, J. W., Sauve, Y., Csonka, K., Karoum, F., & Toffano, G. (1991). Recovery of function in spinalized neonatal rats. *Brain Research Bulletin, 1*, 1–4.

Cornog, M. (2004). The decloseting of masturbation? *Journal of Sex Research, 41*(3), 310–313.

Cotterill, R. M. J. (2000). Did consciousness evolve from self-paced probing of the environment, and not from reflexes?. *Brain and Mind, 1*, 283–298.

Cotterill, R. M. J. (2001). Cooperation of the basal ganglia, cerebellum, sensory cerebrum, and hippocampus: Possible implications for cognition, consciousness, intelligence, and creativity. *Progress in Neurobiology, 64*, 1–33.

Cronin, A., & Mandich, M. B. (2005). *Human development and performance throughout the lifespan*. Clifton Park, NY: Thompson Delmar Learning.

Csikszentmihalyi, M. (1997). *Finding flow*. New York: Basic Books.

Driscoll, M. P. (1994). *Psychology of learning for instruction*. Needham Heights, MA: Allyn & Bacon.

Dubbeldam, J. L. (2001). Evolution of play-like behavior and the uncoupling of neural locomotor mechanisms. *Netherlands Journal of Zoology, 51*, 335–346.

Dudek-Shriber, L. (2004). Parent stress in the neonatal intensive care unit and the influence of parent and infant characteristics. *American Journal of Occupational Therapy, 58*, 509–520.

Dunn, W., & Brown, C. (1997). Factor analysis on the Infant/Toddler Sensory Profile from a national sample of young children without disabilities. *American Journal of Occupational Therapy, 51*(7), 490–495.

Erikson, E. (1964). *Childhood and society*. New York: Norton.

Fenelon, V., Casasnovas, B., Simmers, J., & Meyrand, P. (1998). Development of rhythmic pattern generators. *Current Opinion in Neurobiology, 8*, 705–709.

Ferrari, F., Cioni, G., Einspieler, C., Roversi, F., Bos, A., Paolicelli, P., et al. (2002). Cramped synchronized general movements in preterm infants as an early marker for cerebral palsy. *Archives Pediatrics Adolescent Medicine, 156,* 460–467.

Fidler, G. S., & Fidler, J. W. (1978). Doing and becoming: Purposeful action and self-actualization. *American Journal of Occupational Therapy, 32,* 305–310.

Fisher, A., Murry, E., & Bundy, A. (1991). *Sensory integration: Theory and practice.* New York: F. A. Davis.

Freud, S. (1938). *The basic writings of Sigmund Freud.* New York: The Modern Library.

Gesell, A., & Ilg, F. L. (1949). *Child development, an introduction to the study of human growth.* New York: Harper.

Gilfoyle, E., Grady, A., & Moore, J. (1990). *Children adapt* (2nd ed.). NJ: Slack.

Glovinsky, I. (2005). Moral development, self, and identity. *Journal of Developmental & Behavioral Pediatrics, 26*(2), 160.

Grant, Q. R. (1963). *Child psychiatry.* (Proceedings from the 1963 Occupational Therapy Conference; Reprinted by U.S. Department of Health, Education and Welfare, Public Health Service).

Graybiel, A. M. (1997). The basal ganglia and cognitive pattern generators. *Schizophrenia Bulletin, 23,* 459–469.

Grillner, S., Markram, H., DeSchutter, E., Silberberg, G., & LeBeau, F. E. N. (2005). Microcircuits in action—from CPGs to neocortex. *Trends in Neurosciences, 28*(10), 525–533.

Hagberg, B., Hagberg, G., Beckung, E., & Uvebrant, P. (2001). Changing panorama of cerebral palsy in Sweden, VIII. Prevalence and origin in the birth year period 1991–94. *Acta Paediatrics, 90,* 271–277.

Hall, C. (1954). *A primer of Freudian psychology.* New York: New American Library.

Hanft, B. (2002, March). 2010 express addresses children and youth with special needs. *OT Practice, 14.*

Havighurst, R. J. (1972). *Developmental tasks and education* (3rd ed.). New York: David McKay.

Hess, C. R., Teti, D. M., & Hussey-Gardner, B. (2004). Self-efficacy and parenting of high-risk infants: The moderating role of parent knowledge of infant development. *Journal of Applied Developmental Psychology, 25,* 423–438.

Hinojasa, J., & Kramer, P. (1993). Developmental perspective: Fundamentals of developmental theory. In P. Kramer & J. Hinojosa. (Eds.), *Frames of reference for pediatric occupational therapy,* (pp. 3–8). Baltimore: Williams & Wilkins.

Hunter, J. (2005). Neonatal intensive care unit. In J. Case-Smith (Ed.), *Occupational therapy for children,* (5th ed., pp. 688–770). St Louis: Mosby.

Humphry, R. (2005). Model of processes transforming occupations: Exploring societal and social influences. *Journal of Occupational Science, 12*(1), 36–44.

Jacobs, B. L., & Fornal, C. A. (1997). Seratonin and motor activity. *Current Opinion in Neurobiology, 7,* 820–825.

Johansson, R. S. (1998). Sensory input and control of grip. *Novartis Foundation Symposium, 218*, 45–59.

Kandel, E. R. (2006). *In search of memory*. New York: W. W. Norton.

Kandel, E. R., Schwartz, J. H., & Jessell, T. M. (1995). *Essentials of neural science and behavior*. Stanford, CT: Appleton & Lange.

Kegan, R. (1982). *The evolving self: Problem and process in human development*. Cambridge, MA.: Harvard University Press.

Kemenes, G., Staras, K., & Benjamin, P. R. (2001). Multiple types of control by identified interneurons in a sensory activated rhythmic motor pattern. *The Journal of Neuroscience, 21*, 2903–2911.

Kemenes, I., Straub, V. A., Nikitin, E. S., Staras, K., O'Shea, M., Kemenes, G., et al. (2006). Role of delayed nonsynaptic neuronal plasticity in long term associative memory. *Current Biology, 16*, 1–11.

Kiehn, O., & Kullander, K. (2004). Central pattern generators deciphered by molecular genetics. *Neuron, 41*, 317–321.

King, L. J. (1978). Toward a science of adaptive responses. *American Journal of Occupational Therapy, 32*, 14–22.

Korn, H., & Faure, P. (2003). Is there chaos in the brain? Experimental evidence and related models. *Competes Rendus Biologies, 326*, 787–840.

Kuhle, S., Klebermass, K., Olischar, M., Hulek, M., Prusa, A. R., Kohlhauser, C., et al. (2001). Sleep-wake cycles in preterm infants below 30 weeks of gestational age. Preliminary results of a prospective amplitude integrated EEG study. *Wien Klin Wochenschr, 1*(13), 219–223.

Kuo, A. D. (2002). The relative roles of feedforward and feedback in the control of rhythmic movements. *Motor Control, 6*, 129–145.

Kyler, P., & Merryman, M. B. (2000, November). Healthy people 2010. *OT Practice*, CE-1 to CE-6.

Law, M., Cooper, B., Strong, S., Stewart, S., Rigby, P., & Letts, L. (1996). The person-environment-occupational model: A transactive approach to occupational performance. *Canadian Journal of Occupational Therapy, 63*, 9–23.

Lewis, D. A. (1997). Schizophrenia and disordered neural circuitry. *Schizophrenia Bulletin, 3*, 529–531.

Lewis, Caldwell, & Barker (2003). Modern therapeutic approaches in Parkinson's disease. *Expert Reviews in Molecular Medicine, 5*(10), 1–20.

Littman, B., & Parmelee Jr, A. H. (1978). Medical correlates of infant development. *Pediatrics, 61*(3), 470.

Llorens, L. A. (1966). Aspects of pre-vocational evaluation with psychiatric patients. *Canadian Journal Occupational Theapy, 33*, 5–14.

Llorens, L. A. (1967a). An evaluation procedure for children 6–10 years of age. *American Journal of Occupational Therapy, 21*, 64–69.

Llorens, L. A. (1967b). Projective technique in occupational therapy. *American Journal of Occupational Therapy, 21*, 226–229.

Llorens, L. A. (1968). Changing methods in treatment of psychosocial dysfunction. *American Journal of Occupational Therapy, 22*, 26–29.

Llorens, L. A. (1970). Facilitating growth and development: The promise of occupational therapy. 1969 Eleanor Clarke Slagle Lecture. *American Journal of Occupational Therapy, 24,* 93–101.

Llorens, L. A. (1971). Occupational therapy in community child health. *American Journal of Occupational Therapy, 25,* 335–339.

Llorens, L. A. (1972). Problem-solving the role of occupational therapy in a new environment. *American Journal of Occupational Therapy, 26,* 234–238.

Llorens, L. A. (1973). Activity analysis for cognitive-perceptual-motor dysfunction. *American Journal of Occupational Therapy, 27,* 453–456.

Llorens, L. A. (1975). Occupational therapy consultation in programs for children. *Canadian Journal Occupational Therapy, 41,* 114–117.

Llorens, L. A. (1976). *Application of a developmental theory for health and rehabilitation.* Rockville, MD: American Occupational Therapy Association.

Llorens, L. A. (1977a). A developmental theory revisited. *American Journal of Occupational Therapy, 31,* 656–657.

Llorens, L. A. (1977b). Sequential client care record. *American Journal of Occupational Therapy,* 367–371.

Llorens, L. A. (1981a). On the meaning of activity in occupational therapy. *Journal of the New Zealand Association of Occupational Therapists, 32,* 3–6.

Llorens, L. A. (1981b). *Occupational therapy: State of the art-potential for development.* Paper presented at the New Zealand Association of Occupational Therapists, Inc. Auckland, New Zealand.

Llorens, L. A. (1984a). Changing balance: Environment and individual. *American Journal of Occupational Therapy, 38,* 29–34.

Llorens, L. A. (1984b). Theoretical conceptualizations of occupational therapy, 1960–1982. *Occupational Therapy in Mental Health, 4,* 1–13.

Llorens, L. A. (1986). Activity analysis: Agreement among factors in a sensory processing model. *American Journal of Occupational Therapy, 40,* 103–110.

Llorens, L. A. (1991). Performance tasks and roles throughout the lifespan. In C. Christiansen & C. Baum. (Eds.), *Occupational therapy: Overcoming human performance deficits,* (pp. 45–66). Thorofare, NJ: Charles B. Slack.

Llorens, L. A. (1993). Activity analysis: Agreement between participants and observers on perceived factors in occupation components. *The Occupational Therapy Journal of Research, 13,* 198–211.

Llorens, L. A. (1997a). Forward. In D. E. Watson (Ed.), *Task analysis: An occupational performance approach* (pp. 7–8). Bethesda, MD: The American Occupational Therapy Association.

Llorens, L. A. (1997b). Forward. In G. Gilkerson (Ed.), *Occupational therapy leadership* (pp. 5–6). Philadelphia: F. A. Davis.

Llorens, L. A. (1999). Achieving occupational role: Accommodations for students with disabilities. *Occupational Therapy in Health Care, 11,* 1–8.

Llorens, L. A. (2004). *A fifty-five year odyssey of body, mind, and spirit.* Unpublished Manuscript, pp. 1–15.

Llorens, L. A., & Adams, S. P. (1978). Learning style preferences of occupational therapy students. *American Journal of Occupational Therapy, 32,* 161–164.

Llorens, L. A., & Bernstein, S. P. (1963). Fingerpainting with an obsessive-compulsive organically damaged child. *American Journal of Occupational Therapy, 17,* 120–121.

Llorens, L. A., & Donaldson, K. (1983). Documentation of occupational therapy services: A process model. *Canadian Journal Occupational Therapy, 50,* 171–175.

Llorens, L. A., & Johnson, P. A. (1966). Occupational therapy in an ego-oriented milieu. *American Journal of Occupational Therapy, 20,* 178–181.

Llorens, L. A., Levy, R., & Rubin, E. Z. (1964). Work adjustment program. A prevocational experience. *American Journal of Occupational Therapy, 18,* 15–19.

Llorens, L. A., & Rubin, E. Z. (1962). A directed activity program for disturbed children. *American Journal of Occupational Therapy, 16,* 287–290.

Llorens, L. A., & Rubin, E. Z. (1967). *Developing ego functions in disturbed children.* Detroit, MI: Wayne State University Press.

Llorens, L. A., Rubin, E. Z., Braun, J. S., Beck, G. R., & Beall, C. D. (1969). The effects of a cognitive-perceptual-motor training approach on children with behavior maladjustment. *American Journal of Occupational Therapy, 23,* 502–512.

Llorens, L. A., Rubin, E. Z., Braun, J., Beck, G., Mottley, N., & Beall, D. (1964). Cognitive-perceptual-motor functions. A preliminary report on training. *American Journal of Occupational Therapy, 18,* 202–208.

Llorens, L. A., & Shuster, J. J. (1977). Occupational therapy sequential client care recording system: A comparative study. *American Journal Occupational Therapy, 31*(6), 367–371.

Llorens, L. A., & Young, G. G. (1960). Fingerpainting for the hostile child. *American Journal of Occupational Therapy, 14,* 306–307.

Lydic, R. (1989). Central pattern-generating neurons and the search for general principles. *Federation of American Societies for Experimental Biology, 13,* 2457–2468.

MacLean, P. D. (1973). *A triune concept of the brain and behaviour.* Ontario Mental Health Foundation: University of Toronto Press.

Maier, H. W. (1978). *Three theories of child development* (3rd ed.) New York: Harper and Row.

Majnemer, A. (1998). Benefits of early intervention for children with developmental disabilities. *Seminars in Pediatric Neurology, 5,* 62–69.

Majnemer, A. (2007). Motor incoordination in children born preterm: Coordinated efforts needed. *Developmental Medicine and Child Neurology, 47*(5), 324.

Majnemer, A., & Rosenblatt, B. (1995). Prediction of outcome at school entry in neonatal intensive care unit survivors, with use of clinical and electrophysiologic techniques. *Journal of Pediatrics, 127,* 823–830.

Majnemer, A., Rosenblatt, B., & Riley, R. (1994). Predicting outcome in high risk newborns. *American Journal Occupational Therapy, 48,* 723–732.

Marder, E., & Bucher, D. (2001). Central pattern generators and the control of rhythmic movements. *Current Biology, 11,* 986–996.

Merriam-Webster. (2005). Online. Retrieved January, 10, 2005, from (www.Merriam-Webster.com).

Meyer, A. (1996). The philosophy of occupation therapy. In R. P. Cottrell (Ed.), *Perspectives on purposeful activity: Foundation & future of occupational therapy* (pp. 27–30). Bethesda, MD: American Occupational Therapy Association. (Reprinted from Archives of Occupational Therapy, 1, pp. 1–10, 1921, American Occupational Therapy Association: Bethesda, MD).

Mitcham, M. (2003). Integrating theory and practice: Using theory creatively to enhance professional practice. In G. Brown, S. A. Esdaile, & S. E. Ryan. (Eds.), *Becoming an advanced healthcare practitioner* (pp. 64–89). Boston: Butterworth-Heinemann.

Mosey, A. C. (1974). An alternative: The biopsychosocial model. *American Journal of Occupational Therapy, 28*, 137–140.

Mosey, A. C. (1986). *Psychosocial components of occupational therapy.* New York: Raven.

Mosey, A. C. (1992). *Applied scientific inquiry in the health professions: An epidemological orientation.* Rockville, MD: American Occupational Therapy Association.

Nelson, C. (2001). Cerebral palsy. In D. A. Umphred (Ed.), *Neurological rehabilitation* (4th ed., pp. 259–286). St. Louis, MI: Mosby.

Nelson, D. L. (1986). Occupation: Form and performance. *American Journal of Occupational Therapy, 42*, 633–641.

Olson, J. A., & Baltman, K. (1995). Infant mental health in occupational therapy practice in the neonatal intensive care unit. *The American Journal of Occupational Therapy, 8*, 48–52.

Oppenheim, R. (1984). Ontogenetic adaptations in neural and behavioral development: Toward a more ecological developmental psychobiology. In H. F. R. Prechtl (Ed.), *Continuity of neural functions, from prenatal to post natal life* (pp. 16–30). London: Spastics International Medical Publications.

Paneth, N., & Kiely, J. (1984). *The frequency of cerebral palsy: A review of population studies in industrialized nations since 1950. The epidemiology of the cerebral palsies* (pp. 57–68). London: Heinemann Medical Books.

Papalia, D. E., & Olds, S. W. (1986). *Human development.* New York: McGraw-Hill.

Papalia, D. E., Olds, S. W., & Feldman, R. D. (2001). *Human development* (8th ed.). Boston: McGraw Hill.

Parham, L. D. (1987). Toward professionalism: The reflective therapist. *American Journal of Occupational Therapy, 41*, 555–561.

Parkes, J., Dolk, H., Hill, N., & Pattenden, S. (2001). Cerebral palsy in Northern Ireland: 1981–1993. *Paediatric Perinatology and Epidemiology, 3*, 278–286.

Pearce, J., & Newton, S. (1963)). *Conditions of human growth.* New York: Citadel Press.

Pearson, K. G. (2000). Neural adaptation in the generation of rhythmic behavior. *Annual Review of Physiology, 62*, 723–753.

Peck, R. F., & Havighurst, R. J. (1960)). *The psychology of character development.* New York: Wiley.

Piaget, J. (1952). *The origins of intelligence in children.* (M. Cook, Trans.). New York: International Universities Press.

Prechtl, H. (1997). Editorial: State of the art of a new functional assessment of the young nervous system. An early predictor of cerebral palsy. *Early Human Development, 50,* 1–11.

Prechtl, H. (2001). General movement assessment as a method of developmental neurology: New paradigms and their consequences. *Developmental Medicine & Child Neurology, 43,* 836–842.

Prechtl, H. F. R., & Nolte, R. (1984). Motor behavior in preterm infants. In H. F. R. Prechtl (Ed.), *Continuity of neural functions from prenatal to postnatal life* (pp. 79–93). Oxford: Blackwell Scientific Publications.

Prochazka, A. (1993). Comparison of natural and artificial control of movement. *IEEE Transactions on Rehabilitation Engineering, 1*(1), 7–17.

Reed (1998). Theory and frame of reference. In M. Neistadt & E. Crepeau (Eds.), *Willard & Spackman's occupational therapy* (9th ed., pp. 521–524). Philadelphia: Lippincott.

Reddihough, D. S., & Collins, K. J. (2003). The epidemiology and causes of cerebral palsy. *Australian Journal Physiotherapy, 49,* 7–12.

Redgrave, P., Prescott, T. J., & Gurney, K. (1999). The basal ganglia: A vertebrate solution to the selection problem?. *Neuroscience, 89,* 1009–1023.

Robertson, C. M., Svenson, L. W., & Joffres, M. R. (1998). Prevalence of cerebral palsy in Alberta. *Canadian Journal Neurological Science, 25,* 117–122.

Robertson, C. M., Watt, M. J., & Yasui, Y. (2007). Changes in the prevalence of cerebral palsy for children born very prematurely within a population-based program over 30 years. *Journal American Medical Association, 297*(24), 2733–2740.

Rosenberg, A. (2000). *Philosophy of science: A contemporary introduction.* New York: Routledge.

Royeen, C. (2003). Chaotic occupational therapy: Collective wisdom for a complex profession, 2003 Elanor Clark Slagle lecture. *American Journal of Occupational Therapy, 57,* 609–634.

Sajaniemi, N., Mäkelä, J., Salokorpi, T., von Wendt, L., Hämäläinen, T., & Hakamies-Blomqvist, L. (2001). Cognitive performance and attachment patterns at four years of age in extremely low birth weight infants after early intervention. *European Child & Adolescent Psychiatry, 10,* 122–129.

Schellenburg, J. (1978). *Masters of social psychology.* New York: Oxford University Press.

Schultz, S., & Schkade, J. (1992a). Occupational adaptation: Toward a holistic approach for contemporary practice, part 1. *American Journal of Occupational Therapy, 46,* 829–837.

Schultz, S., & Schkade, J. (1992b). Occupational adaptation: Toward a holistic approach for contemporary practice, part 2. *American Journal of Occupational Therapy, 46,* 917–925.

Silberzahn, M. (March, 1978). Sensory integration theory course based upon the work of A. J. Ayres. Ft. Collins, Colorado.

Sroufe, L. A., Cooper, R. G., & DeHart, G. B. (1996). *Child development: Its nature and course.* New York: McGraw-Hill.

Stanley, F., Blair, E., & Alberman, E. (2000). *Cerebral palsies: Epidemiology & causal pathways.* London: MacKieth Press.

Staras, K., Kemenes, I., Benjamin, P. R., & Kemenes, G. (2003). Loss of self-inhibition is a cellular mechanism for episodic rhythmic behavior. *Current Biology, 13,* 116–124.

Surveillance of Cerebral Palsy in Europe (SCPE). (2000). Surveillance of cerebral palsy in Europe: A collaboration of cerebral palsy surveys and registers. *Developmental Medicine Child Neurology, 42,* 816–824.

Surveillance of Cerebral Palsy in Europe (SCPE). (2002). Prevalence and characteristics of children with cerebral palsy in Europe. *Developmental Medicine and Child Neurology, 44,* 633–640.

Thelen, E. (1995). Motor development: A new synthesis. *American Psychologist, 50*(2), 79–95.

Touwen, B. C. (1984). Primitive reflexes-conceptual or semantic problem?. In H. F. R. Prechtl (Ed.), *Continuity of neural functions, from prenatal to post natal life* (pp. 115–124). Oxford: Blackwell Scientific Publications.

United Nations. (2002). *Convention on the rights of the child.* Geneva: Author.

United States Department of Health, Education, and Welfare. (1980). *Promoting health/preventing disease: Objectives for the nation.* Washington, DC: U.S. Government Printing Office.

United States Department of Health, Education, and Welfare. (1990). *Healthy people 2000: National health promotion and disease prevention objectives.* (PHS Publication No. 91–50213). Washington, DC: U.S. Government Printing Office.

United States Department of Health, Education, and Welfare. (2001). Healthy people 2010: Understanding and improving health. Retrieved November 19, 2001, from http://www.usmc-mccs.org/semperfit/fithlth/healthypeople2010/html/volume2/16mich Htm#_toc94699666

von Holst, E. (1973). *The behavioral physiology of animal and man: The collected books of Erich von Holst* (Vol. 1). London: Methuen.

Waite, T. (2003). *Activity theory.* Retrieved Dec. 12, 2004, Indiana University, from http://www.slis.indiana.edu/faculty/yrogers/act_theory2/

Walker, K., & Shortridge, S. D. (1993). Lela Llorens. In R. Miller & K. Walker (Eds.), *Perspectives on theory for the practice of occupational therapy.* Frederick, MD: Aspen Publishers.

West, W. (1984). A reaffirmed philosophy and practice of occupational therapy for the 1980s. *The American Journal of Occupational Therapy, 38,* 15–34.

Whitley, S., & Cowan, M. (1991). Developmental intervention in the newborn intensive care unit. *NAACOG's Clinical Issues in Perinatal and Women's Health Nursing, 2,* 84–110.

Wilcock, A. A. (1999). Reflections on doing, being and becoming. *Australian Occupational Therapy Journal, 46,* 1–11.

Wilson-Costello, D., Friedman, H., Minich, N., Fanaroff, A. A., & Hack, M. (2005). Improved survival rates with increased neuro-developmental disability for extremely low birth weight infants in the 1990s. *Pediatrics, 115*(4), 997–1003.

Winkelmann, R. K. (1959). *The erogenous zones: Their nerve supply and significance.* http://www.cirp.org/library/anatomy/winkelmann/ (Vol. 34, pp. 39–47). Mayo Clinic Proceedings (File revised September 11, 2004).

Winter, S., Autry, A., Boyle, C., & Yeargin-Allsopp, M. (2002). Trends in the prevalence of cerebral palsy in a population based study. *Pediatrics, 110*, 1220–1225.

World Health Organization. (1986). *Definition: Health promotion.* Geneva: Author.

World Health Organization. (2001). *International classification of functioning, disability, and health (icf).* Geneva: World Health Organization.

Wright, K. (2004). Times of our lives. *Scientific American, Special Edition, 14*, 42–49.

y Ribotta, M. G., Provencher, J., Feraboli-Lohnherr, D., Rossignol, S., Privat, A., & Orsal, D. (2000). Activation of locomotion in adult chronic spinal rats is achieved by transplantation of embryonic raphe cells reinnervating a precise lumbar level. *The Journal of Neuroscience, 20*, 5144–5152.

Yerxa, E. J. (1996). Dreams, dilemmas and decisions for O.T. practice in a new millennium: An American perspective. In R. P. Cottrell (Ed.), *Perspectives on purposeful activity: Foundation & future of occupational therapy* (pp. 613–616). Bethesda, MD: American Occupational Therapy Association. (Reprinted from *American Journal of Occupational Therapy, 48*, pp. 586–589, 1994).

Yuste, R., MacLean, J. N., Smith, J., & Lansner, A. (2005). The cortex as a central pattern generator. *Nature Reviews Neuroscience, 6*(6), 477–484.

Zehr, E. P., Carroll, T. J., Chua, R., Collins, D. F., Frigon, A., Haridas, C., et al. (2004). Possible contributions of central pattern generator activity to the control of rhythmic human arm movement. *Canadian Journal Physiological Pharmacology, 82*, 556–568.

Zigler, E. P., & Valentine, J. (Eds.). (1979). *Project head start: A legacy of the war on poverty.* New York: Free Press.

APPENDIX A

Models of (1) Johansson (1998), (2) Llorens (1991), and (3) Silberzahn (March, 1978).

Model 1 Depicts the Predictive CPG "Feed-Forward" of Sensation for Grip.

MODEL 1. From Johansson, R. S. (1998) (reproduced with permission). The Role of Sensory Input in the Control of Grip is Illustrated. The Specific Properties of the Task are Contrasted Against the Sensorimotor Action Programs that Represent Procedural Memories. The Anticipatory Control Parameter Indicates the Expected, While the Specific Use of Sensory Information for Corrective Measures is Termed Discrete Event, Sensory Driven Control

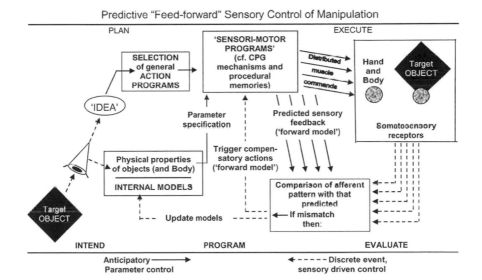

Model 2 Provides a Rationale for the Use of Occupation.

MODEL 2. From Llorens (1991) (reproduced with permission)

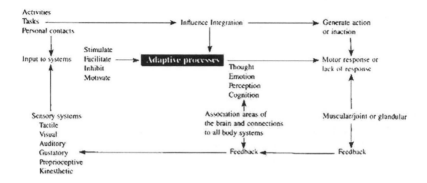

Model 3: For Sensory Integration (SI) Theory.

MODEL 3. From Silberzahn (1978). Also see Ayres (1972)

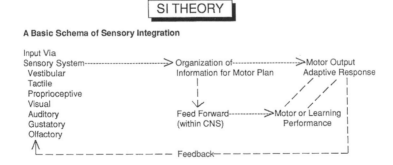

APPENDIX B. Schematic Representation of Achieving Growth and Development

Section 1 - Part 1
Developmental Expectations, Behaviors and Needs
(Occupational Enablement)

Sensorimotor		Physical-Motor	Psychosocial
Neuropsychological (Ayres)	Occupational Physiology *(Moore, von Holt)*	(Gesell)	(Erikson)
0-2 yrs. Sensorimotor; Tactile, vestibular, visual, auditory, olfactory, gustatory functions	*Central Pattern Generator: A-M System: 2wks GA-10 yrs.: Homeostatic, circadian rhythms, endocrine funct., attention, orientation time/ space; spatian, movements*	0-2 yrs. Head sags, Fisting; Gross motion, Walking, Climbing	Basic Trust vs. Mistrust/Oral; Sensory: Ease of feeding; Depth of sleep; Relax. of bowels
6 mo.-4 yrs Integration of Body Sides; Gross motor plan, Form & space, Balance; Post. and bilateral integration; Body scheme develop.	*Central Pattern Generator: Paer System: 5 mos. GA-7 yrs. Enet. reg. + latency; patterns of locomotor affective responses; orientation, visual, auditory, and somatosensory; protection*	2-3 yrs. Runs; Balances; Hand preference; Coordination	Autonomy vs. Shame & Doubt/ Muscular-Anal; Conflict between holding on & letting go
3-7; Discrimination; Refined tactile, kinesth, visual, auditory, olfact., gustatory functions	*Central Pattern Generator: Neocortical System: 8 mos. GA-maturity: Exploratory/ discriminative, skillful, information integration, creat'n/cart., motor phonic-g/semi-automatic movements.*	3-6 yrs. Coordination more graceful; Muscles develop; Skills develop	Initiative vs. Guilt/Locomotor-Genital; Aggressiveness; Manipulation; Coercion
(delete 3-; change to 6-8 yrs. -) Abstract Thinking; Conceptualization; Complex relations; Read, write numbers	*Central Pattern Generator: Neo-Neo System: Birth-maturity: self reflect. /judgment emotional stability, motivation; memory circuits, semantics*	6-11 yrs. Energy development; Skill practice to attain proficiency	Industry vs. Inferiority/Latency; Wins recognition thru productivity; Learns skills & tools
Continue to develop; Conceptualization; Complex relations; Read, write numbers	*Central Pattern Generation is neurochemically emergent and distinctive throughout Arch/Paleo/Neo and Neo-Neo systems for Occupational Performance (stimuli association, selection processing/engagement)*	11-13 yrs. Rapid growth; Poor posture; Awkwardness	Identity vs. Role Confusion/Puberty & Adolescence; Identification; Social Roles
Development presumably maintained	*These dynamic systems work together, and exhibit variability in their complexity*	Growth established and maintained	Intimacy vs. Isolation/Young Adulthood; Commitments; Body & ego mastery
Alterations begin to occur in sensory functions, conceptualization, and memory		Alterations begin to occur in motor behavior, strength, and endurance	Generativity vs. Stagnation/Adulthood; Guiding next generation; Creative, productive
Alterations in sensory functions, conceptualization, and memory		Alterations in motor behavior, strength and endurance	Ego Integrity vs. Despair/Maturity; Acceptance of own life cycle

Ecology of the Microsystem (Bronfenbrenner, 1979). Provide: dynamic opportunities for Spatiotemporal tortogenetic Adaptation, or occupational enablement, in the meso, exo and macrosystem spheres of growth and development.

Note: Adapted from Llorens (1991, p. 48-49). Applied changes are Italicized.

APPENDIX B. Continued

Section 1 – Part 2
Developmental Expectations, Behaviors and Needs
(Occupational Enablement)

Psychodynamic

Psychosexual	Character Development
Object-Affect-Action Erogenous Zone Development ; *(Freud) (as discussed by Freud/Growth/Hall)*	*(Peck/Havinghurst)*
0-4 yrs. <u>Oral Zone</u> Dependency Init. Aggress; *object cathexes with breast/bottle, thumb/pacifier;* *Genital erogenous zone arousal and coaterotism.*	**Infancy: <u>Amoral Type</u>** *Follows whims and impulses* *Self gratification* *Lacks internal moral prin, conscious, or superego*
0-4 yrs. <u>Anal-sadistic Zone</u>: *Autoervsion increases with sphincter control;* Independence, Resistiveness, Self-assertiveness Narcissism Ambivalence; *Genital masturbation is cyclic and oscillating, interspersed with latency* *Eyes: visual exploration, "looking" discrimination.*	
3-6 yrs. Delete *(Genital-Oedipal Genital interest Poss. of opp. parent, antag. to same parent. Castration fears)* <u>Phallic Zone</u>: *Social Experience (oedipal object relations) pivotal in character Development;* Deep affection for Opposite sex parent , authority: Struggle/identification same sex parent, genital masturbation and sphincter coordination. *Eyes: Visual exploration "looking" at playmates and adult genitalia, obser. toileting. Knowledge subline. For investigation.*	**Early Childhood:** **Expedient type:** *Self-Centered, conscience and superego not consistently rational; needs external controls to guide behavior*
6-11 yrs. *Latency or Partial Latency due to sexual inhibition,* (Oedetx-Prim. struggles quiescent) *Genital masturbation may be suppressed, or continue. Eyes identify object attractors;* Init. in mastery of skills. Strong defenses.	**6-13 yrs. Either of these types:** *Conforming: Role bound behavior; consequences not relevant. Crude conscience* *Irrational Conscientious: Follows A set of internalized ideals: rigid superego; disregards effects of actions on others.*
11- Adolescence <u>Genital Zone Maturation</u>: *Ability for privacy.* Breasts: (women) mature as erogenous zone and attractor. Eyes: Visual excitement of sexual objects (images, symbols) Emancip. from parents Occup. decisions Role experiment Re-exam of Values	**13- Rational – Altruistic:** *Uses judgment to guide interpersonal activities; Consideration of others as much as consideration of self. Ongoing dev. Throughout life span.*
Outgrow need for parent validation; identify with others, selection of love object, sexual aims, and sublimation of sexual energy for creativity:	Give and receive love; productive endeavors (Adler & Jung, as discussed by Berger, 2000, Peck & Havighurst, 1960; Schellenburg, 1978)
Emotional responsibilities may lessen Phys. and econ. indepdend. Accepted Shift from survival to enjoyment	
Continued growth after middle age Inner trend toward survival	

Ecology of the Microsystem (Bronfenbrenner, 1979). Provides dynamic opportunities for spatiotemporal (ontogenetic) adaptation, or occupational enablement, in the meso, exo and macrosystem spheres of growth and development.

Note: Adapted from Llorens (1991, p. 48-49). Applied changes are italicized.

APPENDIX B. Continued

Section 1 – Part 3
Developmental Expectations, Behaviors and Needs
(Occupational Enablement)

Sociocultural (Gesell)	Social (Cognitive) Language		Social Cognition & Self-efficacy (Bandura)	Activity of Daily Living (Gesell)
	Language (Gesell)			
Oral erotic activity Individual –mothering person most important Immediate - family group important	Small sounds Coos Vocalizes Listens Speaks		*Infancy* *Obs Learning* *Percept. conseq. of actions–diff. self from others*	Recognizes bottle Holds spoon Holds glass Controls bowel
Parallel play Often alone Recognizes extended family	Identifies objects verb. Asks "why?" Short sentences		*Early Childhood: Anticipatory behavior results from family, school and peer relationships*	Feeds self Helps undress Recognizes simple tunes No longer wets at night
Seeks companionship Makes decisions Plays with other children Takes turns	Combines talking and eating Complete sentences Imaginative Dramatic			Laces shoes Cuts with scissors Toilets independently Helps set table
Group play & team activities Independence of adults Gang interests	Language major form of communication		*7-12 yrs.* *Opportunities for creativity;* *Self-rating of progress in meeting goals. Cognitive capacities challenged*	Enjoys dressing up Learns value of money Responsible for grooming
Team games Organization important Interest in opposite sex	Verbal language predominates		*Adolescence:* *Symbolic modeling by peers, teachers and parents results in antecedent behavior*	Interest in earning money
Group affiliation Family, social, civic interest	Non-verbal behavior used		*Adulthood* *Occupational choice is determined by self-efficacy beliefs.* *Innovative planning for family and voc adjustments*	Concern for personal grooming, mate, family
			Advancing Age: *Re-eval efficacy for physical and productive activities* *Actions to maintain health efficacy*	Accepting and adjusting to changes of middle age
			Old-Age *Use cognition to compensate for increasing frailty*	Adjusting to changes after middle age

Ecology of the Microsystem (Bronfenbrenner, 1979). Provides dynamic opportunities for spatiotemporal "ontogenetic" adaptation, or occupational enablement, in the meso, exo and macrosystem spheres of growth and development.

Note: Adapted from Llorens (1991, p. 48–49). Applied changes are italicized.

Section 2
Achieving Activities and Relationships (Selected)
(Occupation for Performance in Work/Education, Play/Leisure, Self-care, and Rest/Relaxation Time Activities)

Integrative Sensorimotor Activities (Activation, organization, and *modulation of all central* processing/patterning to all body systems) La Corte, 2004)	Developmental Activities (*Play and learning occupations; skill achievement* (La Corte, 2004; Llorens, 1976))	Symbolic Activities	Daily Life Tasks (*All occupationally vital life tasks; performance in instrumental and daily care [maintenance] activities, Lfk, 2004)*	Interpersonal Activities
Focused: Tactile, visual, aud., olfact., gust., vestibular and proprioceptive input (delete=Stimulation)	Dolls, Animals, Sand, Water, Excursions	Biting, Chewing, Eating, Blowing, Cuddling	Recog. food, Hold feed. equip., Use feed. equip.	Individual interaction *(Dyadic Reciprocity according to Bronfenbrenner, 1979)*
Phys. positions and exercise, tracking, *posturing, signaling comfort and distress.* Body scheme and image, Postural - ocular control, Discrimination, Balancing, Motor planning	Pull toys, Playground, Clay, Crayons, Chalk	Throwing, Dropping, Messing, Collecting, Destroying	Feeding, Toileting	Individual interaction, Parallel play *(Dyadic and N + 2 systems; according to Bronfenbrenner, 1979)*
Listening, Learning, Skilled tasks & games	Being read to, Coloring, Drawing, Painting	Destroying, Exhibiting	Feeding, Dressing, Toileting, Simple chores	Individual interaction, Play small groups, *Dynamic Group Interaction and Interdependency (Lewin, as described by Schellenburg, 1978)*
Reading, Writing, Numbers	Scooters, Wagons, Collections, Puppets, Bldg.	Controlling, Mastery	Feeding, Dressing, Grooming, Spending	Individual interaction, Groups, Teams, Clubs
All of the above available to be recycled	Weaving, Machinery tasks, Carving, Modeling	All of the above available to be recycled	Feeding, Dressing, Grooming, Pre-voc. skills	Individual interaction, Groups, Teams
	Arts Crafts, Sports Club & interest groups, *Occupational Roles:* *Leisure*, *Education*, *Work*		Feeding, Dressing, Grooming, *Occupational Life role skills (ADL & IADL)*, *Intuition*, *Creativity*, *Insight*	Individual interaction, Groups
	Developmental Mastery for Occupational Enablement	*Purposeful Activities and Dyadic Reciprocity include sensorimotor integration, dev. of appropriate affective responses, and the ability to relate appropriately to objects (Llorens, p. 37) Mesosystem linkages to all other Micro, Exo, and Macro systems. (Bronfenbrenner, 1979)*	*Developmental Mastery for Successful Occupational Role Adaptation*	

Developmental Mastery for Occupational Enablement

Note: Adapted from Llorens (1991, p. 48-49). Applied changes are italicized.

APPENDIX B. Continued

Section 3
Behavior Expectations and Adaptive Skills
(Environmental [physical and socio-cultural] Adaptation)

Developmental Tasks (Havighurst; Peck & Havighurst)	Human Ecology (Bronfenbrenner)	Ego-Adaptive Skills (Mosey; Pearce & Newton)	Discovery Learning through Play and Scaffolding (Bruner)	Intellectual Development (Piaget)
Learning to walk, talk, take solids; Elimination	*Differentiated perception and response; Dyadic change, visual disc. for shapes, mother's voice*	Ability to respond to mothering; Mastering of gross motor responses	*0-3 yrs.: Enactive Stage; Motor learning of action sequences*	Motor skills; Integrated
Sex difference; Form concepts of soc. & physical reality; Relate emotionally to others; Right vs. wrong; Develop a conscience	*Directing and controlling one's own behavior; Enjoys peek-a-boo, cuddling, looking at books, music; saying "no"*	Ability to respond to routines of daily living Mastery of 3 dimen. space; Sense of body image	→	Investigative; Imitative; Egocentric
Symbolic expressions of spirituality; Motivational quest for life's meaning	*Coping successfully under stress. Ecological transitions between Microsystems, generalize objects and relationships to adapt to new contexts.*	Ability to respond to routines of daily living Mastery of 3 dimen. space; Tolerate frustrations; Sit still; Delay gratification	*3-8 yrs: Iconic Stage. Visual memory for concrete objects and relationships stored in categorical schemas*	Egocentrism reduced, social increased; Lang. Rep. motor
Learn phys. skills; Getting along; Reading, writing; Values; Social attitudes	*Acquiring knowledge and skill, didactic activities of the occ. role entail new object relationships*	Ability to perceive, sort, organize & utilize stimuli; Work in groups; Master inanimate obj.	*6-8 yrs - developing through adulthood: Symbolic Stage; Increasingly more diffuse ability for self conscious reflectiveness*	Orders exper.; Relates parts to wholes; Deduct.
More mature relationships; Social roles; Select occupation; Achieving emot. Independence	*Establishing and maintaining mutually rewarding relationships: N+2 systems*	Ability to accept & discharge responsibility; Capacity for love		Systematic approach to problems; Sense of equality; *Induction*
Selecting a mate; Starting a family Marriage, home; Congenial social group	*Modifying and constructing one's own physical, social, and symbolic environment: "power" connections shape policy, funding, politics, and philosophy of culture and subculture.*	Ability to function indep.; Control drives; Plan & execute; Purposeful motions; Obtain org. & use knowledge; Part. in primary group; Part. in variety of relationships; Exp, self as accept.; Part. in mutually satisfying heterosexual relations		Development established and maintained
Civic & social responsibility; Econ. standard of living; Dev. adult leisure activities; Adjust to aging parents; Adjust to decr. phys. health, retire., death; Age group affiliations - Meeting social obligations; *Occupational Self - themes of meaning (Jackson, Llorens)*			*Narrative (Bruner)*	Alterations in other areas may affect

Ecology of the Exosystem system (Bronfenbrenner, 1979) = Occupational (Role) Adaptation: the process of mutual accommodation between the person, their occupational activity, and the changing environment. Incorporates Occupational Readiness (Schultz & Schade, 1992a, 1992, b).

Ecology of the Macrosystem = Prototype of culture and subculture (Bronfenbrenner, 1979); Includes occupational (a) form (object, (Nelson, 1986), (b) socialization (Mead, as discussed by Schellenburg, 1978), (c) performance (Llorens, 1976) and, (d)context (Bronfenbrenner, 1979)

Note: Adapted from Llorens (1991, p. 48-49). Applied changes are italicized.

Index